Eco-Conscious Skincare: A Journey to Radiant Skin and a Healthier Planet

By Celeste Bloom

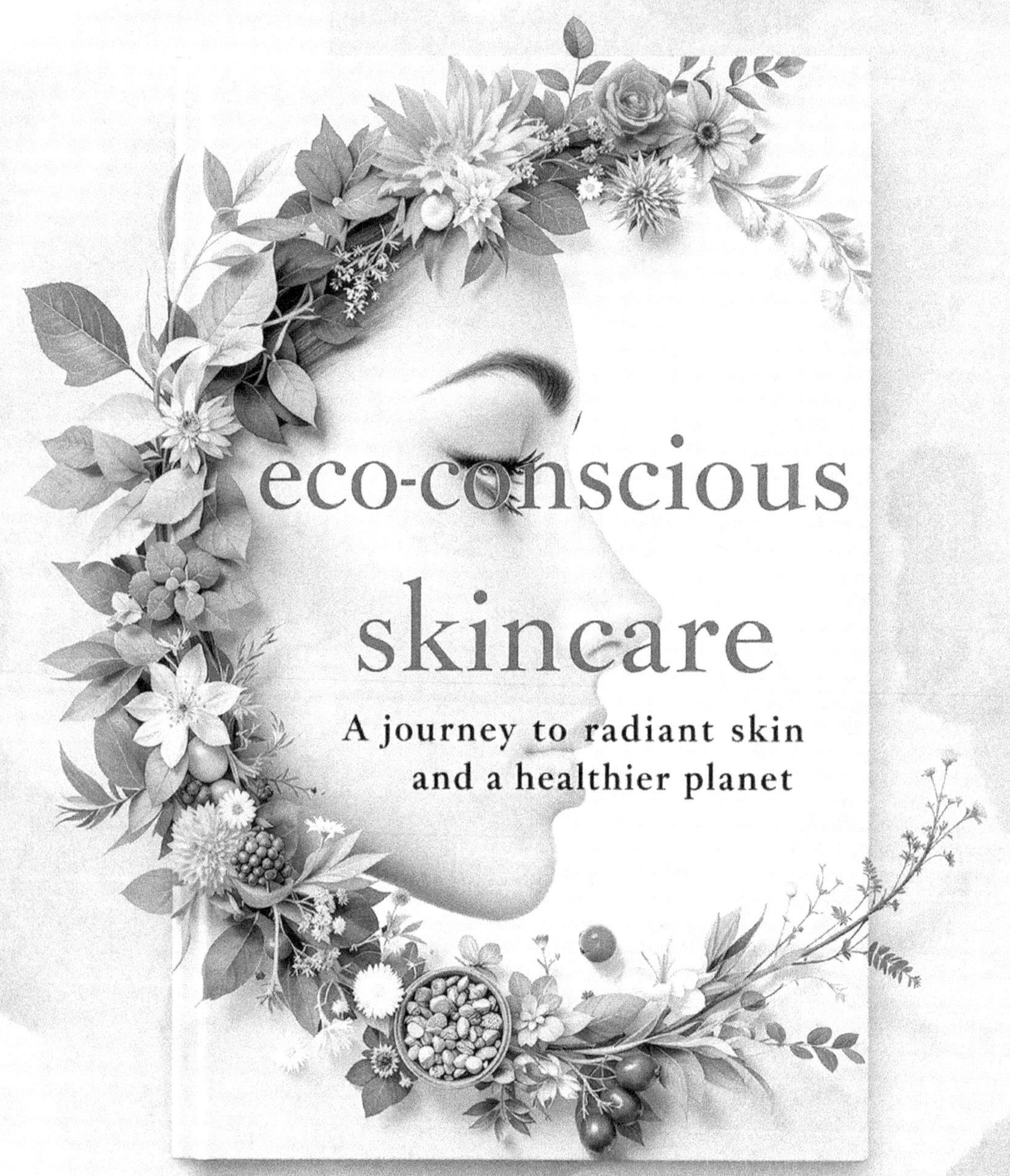

CELESTE BLOOM

Table of Contents

Chapter 4: Sourcing Sustainable Ingredients

Chapter 5: Customizing Your Skincare Routine

Chapter 6: Launching Your Skincare Business

Introduction

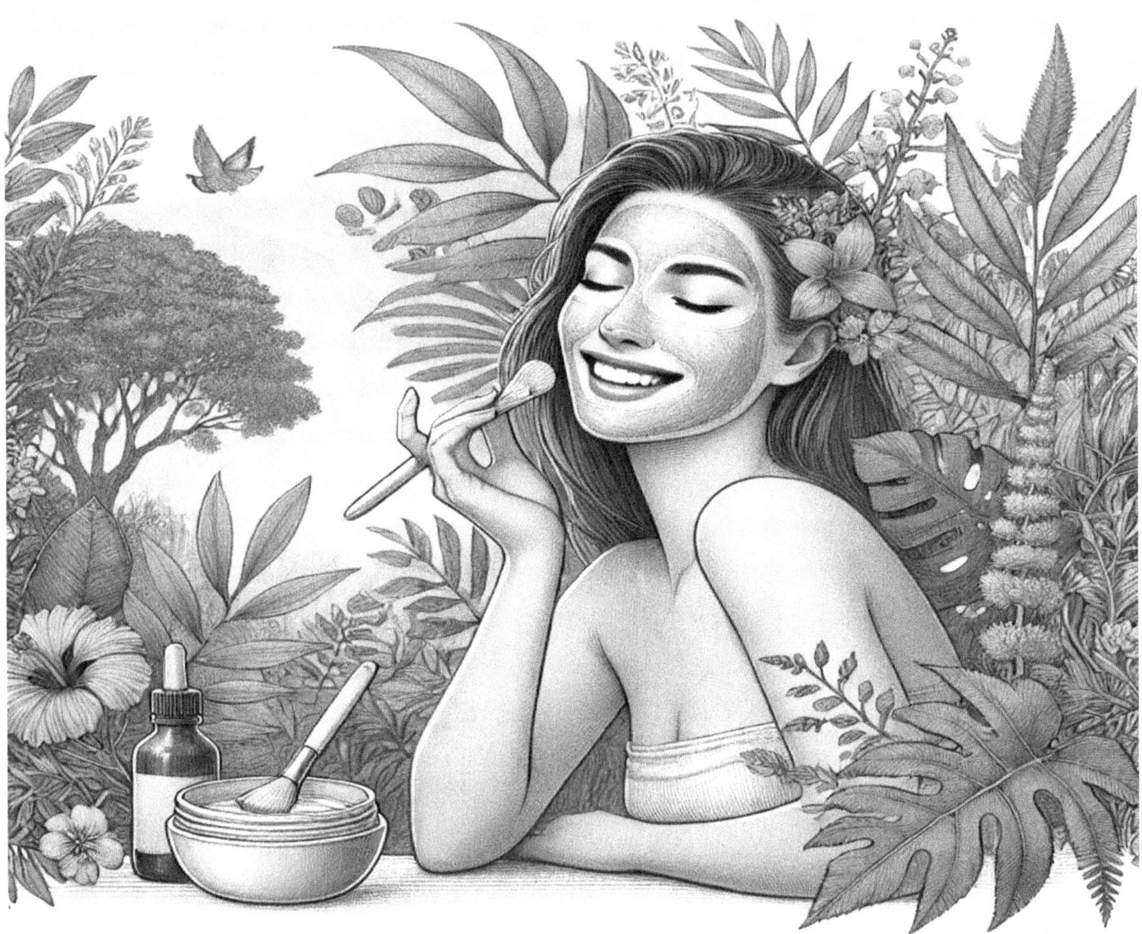

Welcome, dear reader, to this journey of self-discovery and sustainable living. As a woman navigating the complexities of modern life, I've always been drawn to the idea of living in harmony with nature. This fascination led me down a path of exploring natural remedies and, eventually, the world of DIY skincare. What began as a personal quest for healthier skin blossomed into a deeper understanding of the interconnectedness between our well-being, our choices, and the planet we inhabit.

This book is a culmination of my experiences, research, and passion for creating a more sustainable and fulfilling life. It's a guide for women like you who are seeking a holistic approach to beauty, one that nourishes both your skin and the environment. We'll delve into the science behind healthy skin, explore the art of formulating natural skincare products, and discover how to make conscious choices that benefit both you and the planet.

Remember, this is not just a book about skincare; it's an invitation to embark on a transformative journey of self-care, sustainability, and empowerment. Let's embrace the power of nature, nurture our skin, and contribute to a healthier planet, one conscious choice at a time.

Chapter 1: The Journey to Eco-Friendly Skincare

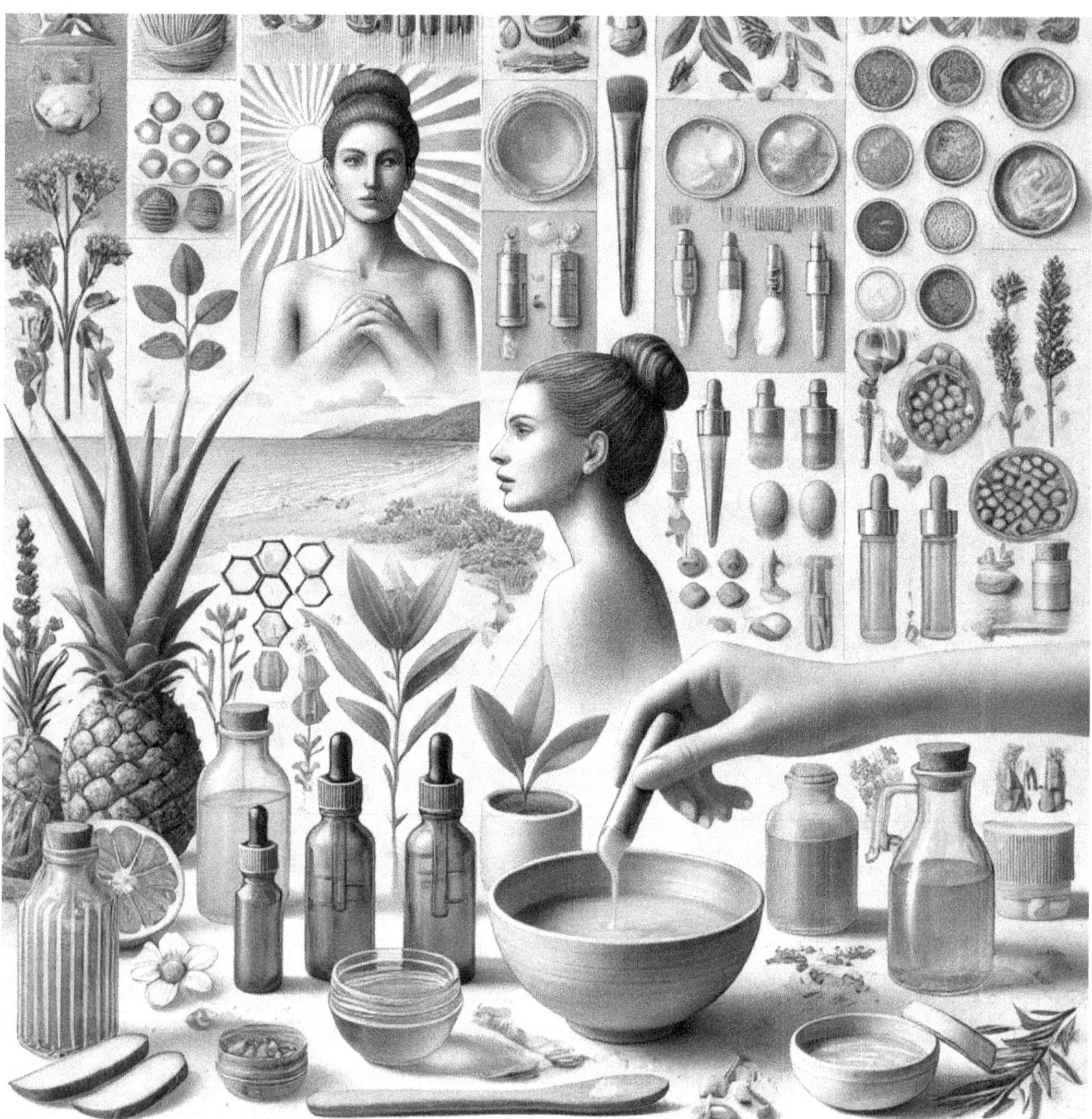

Setting the Stage

I vividly recall the day I stumbled upon a small, unassuming blog dedicated to DIY skincare. Intrigued by the idea of creating my own beauty products, I embarked on a journey that would not only transform my skincare routine but also reshape my understanding of beauty and sustainability. The allure of crafting natural remedies, free from harsh chemicals and artificial fragrances, was undeniable.

A Greener-Healthier Approach

This book explores the profound impact of embracing eco-friendly skincare practices. We'll discover how to create healthier, more effective skincare solutions while minimizing our environmental footprint. By understanding the principles of sustainable living and harnessing the power of nature, we can achieve radiant skin and contribute to a healthier planet.

Supporting Content

Defining Eco-Friendly Skincare: Eco-friendly skincare prioritizes the use of natural, plant-based ingredients, minimizes waste, and supports sustainable practices throughout the product lifecycle. This means choosing products that are free from harmful chemicals like parabens, phthalates, and sulphates, and opting for brands that prioritize ethical sourcing and minimal packaging.

The DIY Advantage: DIY skincare empowers you to control the ingredients, ensuring they align with your values and skin needs. By creating your own products, you can avoid potentially harmful chemicals and tailor your formulations to your specific skin type and concerns. Additionally, DIY skincare reduces reliance on mass-produced products, often packaged in excessive plastic and contributing to environmental waste.

Zero-Waste Principles in Beauty: We'll explore strategies for minimizing waste in your beauty routine, such as:

Refilling containers: Invest in reusable containers and refill them with your DIY creations or purchase products from brands that offer refill options.

Embracing minimalism: Choose multi-purpose products and avoid unnecessary packaging. Opt for products with minimal or recyclable packaging whenever possible.

Composting: Compost any organic waste from your skincare products, such as used tea bags or coffee grounds.

Skincare and Sustainability: Our skin is our largest organ, and what we apply to it directly impacts our health and the environment. By choosing eco-friendly options, we prioritize both personal well-being and planetary health. The chemicals used in conventional skincare products can potentially disrupt our hormone systems and have negative impacts on the environment. By choosing natural, plant-based ingredients, we can minimize our exposure to harmful chemicals and support a healthier planet.

Starting Small - A Beginner's Guide: We'll begin with simple, easy-to-follow recipes and gradually progress to more complex formulations, ensuring a smooth and enjoyable learning experience. Starting with basic recipes like a simple facial oil or a hydrating toner can build confidence and encourage further exploration.

Stories of Inspiration

Anya's Transformation

Anya, a driven professional balancing long hours at work and a hectic city lifestyle, often found herself grappling with persistent skin issues. For years, she struggled with redness, irritation, and sensitivity that conventional skincare products only seemed to exacerbate. Determined to find a solution, Anya began researching the ingredients in her products and was shocked to discover a host of synthetic chemicals and potential irritants.

Her journey into DIY skincare began when a close friend gifted her a homemade calendula-infused balm. The soothing effects were almost immediate, sparking her curiosity about natural remedies. Encouraged, Anya decided to try crafting her own skincare products. She started small, experimenting with simple recipes like a gentle oatmeal cleanser and a hydrating rosewater toner.

As Anya delved deeper into the world of DIY skincare, she not only noticed a dramatic improvement in her skin's health and clarity but also experienced a profound shift in her lifestyle. Embracing natural living, she began sourcing organic ingredients from local farmers' markets and eliminated single-use plastics from her routine. What began as a quest for healthier skin evolved into a holistic approach to sustainable living.

Today, Anya feels more connected to her choices and the planet. She shares her journey through workshops and community events, inspiring others to embrace eco-friendly skincare and natural living. Her transformation demonstrates that small, conscious changes can lead to remarkable, lasting benefits—not just for our skin but for our overall well-being and the environment.

A Global Tapestry of Beauty

Beauty practices rooted in nature have been an integral part of cultures worldwide for centuries, offering a rich tapestry of traditions that honor the relationship between humanity and the environment.

In India, the ancient system of Ayurveda emphasizes balancing the mind, body, and spirit for optimal health, including radiant skin. Ayurvedic beauty treatments often incorporate herbs like turmeric for its anti-inflammatory properties, sandalwood for its cooling effects,

and amla (Indian gooseberry) for its rich antioxidants. These traditions, passed down through generations, showcase the timeless efficacy of natural ingredients.

Across the globe in indigenous North American communities, healing wisdom is deeply intertwined with nature. Ingredients like bearberry, wild rose, and yucca root are used in skincare and healing rituals, symbolizing the interconnectedness of the land and its people. These practices reflect a deep respect for the Earth's resources and the need to use them sustainably.

In Africa, shea butter, often referred to as "women's gold," has been a beauty staple for centuries. Extracted from the nuts of the shea tree, this rich butter is celebrated for its moisturizing and healing properties. Beyond its skincare benefits, the production of shea butter is also a vital economic resource for many rural communities, empowering women and preserving cultural heritage.

In East Asia, countries like Japan and Korea have long embraced the use of fermented ingredients, such as rice water and soybean extract, in their beauty rituals. These elements not only enhance the skin's radiance but also reflect a philosophy of harnessing nature's power through patience and precision.

This global tapestry of natural beauty practices not only underscores the universality of seeking harmony with nature but also highlights the importance of preserving cultural wisdom. These traditions remind us that the path to beauty is not just about external appearances but about respecting the heritage, resources, and knowledge passed down through generations.

Key Takeaway

Embracing eco-friendly skincare is a transformative journey that extends far beyond simply achieving healthy skin. It's a journey of self-discovery and empowerment. By understanding the principles of sustainability, we gain a deeper appreciation for the interconnectedness of our actions and their impact on the environment.

This shift towards conscious consumption empowers us to make informed choices that align with our values and contribute to a healthier planet. By choosing natural, plant-based ingredients, minimizing waste, and supporting sustainable practices, we can create a beauty routine that nourishes both our skin and the environment. This conscious approach not only benefits our individual health and well-being but also contributes to a healthier and more sustainable future for all.

Understanding Your Skin

Before we delve into the world of DIY formulations, let's embark on a fascinating journey within – a journey into the intricate world of skin biology. Just as every snowflake is unique, so is your skin. Understanding its complex structure and functions is crucial for creating a skincare routine that truly nourishes and protects.

This chapter will explore the intricate layers of your skin, from the protective epidermis to the collagen-rich dermis. We'll delve into the fascinating world of skin types, understanding the unique characteristics of oily, dry, combination, and sensitive skin. You'll learn how natural ingredients interact with your skin, from hydrating oils to antioxidant-rich botanicals.

Furthermore, we'll explore the vital role of pH balance in maintaining a healthy skin barrier and discuss how external factors like sun exposure, pollution, and diet can significantly impact your skin's health and appearance. By understanding these key aspects of skin biology, you'll gain the knowledge and confidence to make informed choices about your skincare routine and create personalized solutions that truly address your individual needs.

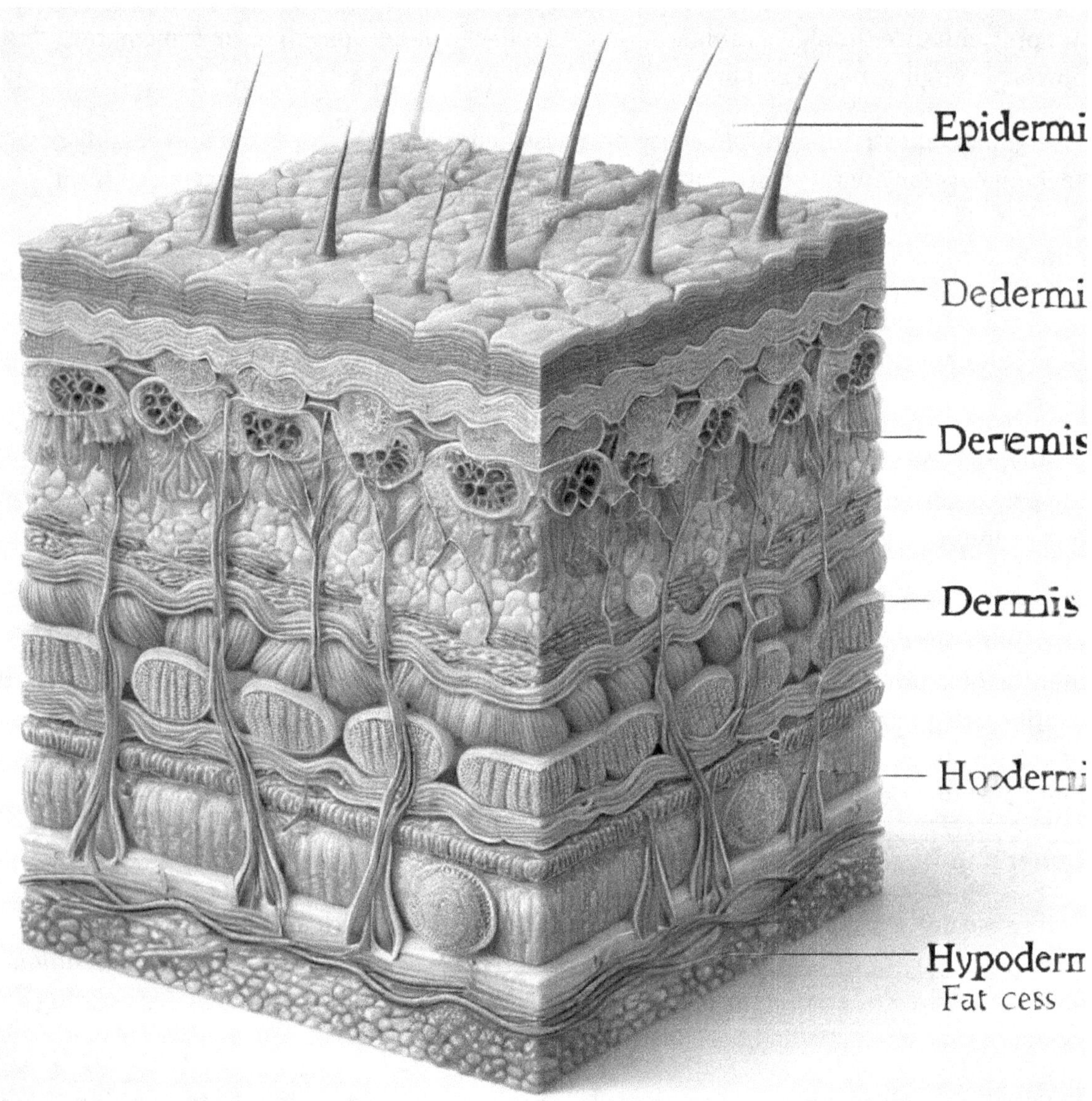

Do You Really Know Your Skin?

Have you ever wondered why certain skincare products work wonders for some and do little for others? The answer lies in understanding the unique biology of your skin. Just as every snowflake is unique, so is your skin.

Unveiling the Mysteries of Your Skin

Anatomy and Physiology: Let's delve deeper into the intricate layers of your skin:

Epidermis: The outermost layer, acting as a protective barrier against external factors.

Dermis: The thickest layer, containing collagen, elastin, and blood vessels that provide nourishment and support.

Hypodermis: The deepest layer, primarily composed of fat cells that provide insulation and cushioning.

Skin Types Demystified: Understanding your skin type is crucial for choosing the right ingredients and formulations. Common skin types include:

Oily skin: Characterized by excess oil production, often leading to shine and breakouts.

Dry skin: Lacks sufficient oil production, resulting in dryness, flakiness, and tightness.

Combination skin: A combination of oily and dry areas, typically with an oily T-zone (forehead, nose, and chin) and dry cheeks.

Sensitive skin: Reacts easily to irritants, often experiencing redness, itching, and stinging.

The Language of Your Skin: Let's explore how natural ingredients interact with your skin:

Hydrators: Ingredients like hyaluronic acid, aloe vera, and glycerine attract and retain moisture, keeping your skin hydrated and plump.

Emollients: Oils like jojoba, argan, and sweet almond oil help to soften and smooth the skin by filling in the gaps between skin cells.

Antioxidants: Vitamin C, vitamin E, and green tea extract protect the skin from environmental damage caused by free radicals.

Exfoliants: Ingredients like AHAs (alpha hydroxy acids) and BHAs (beta hydroxy acids) help to remove dead skin cells, revealing smoother, brighter skin.

pH Balance - The Key to Healthy Skin: Maintaining the optimal pH balance of your skin is essential for a healthy barrier function. The slightly acidic pH of your skin helps to protect against harmful bacteria and maintain a healthy microbiome.

Environmental Influences - A Skin's Story: Learn how factors like sun exposure, pollution, and diet can impact your skin's health and appearance:

Sun exposure: UV radiation from the sun can accelerate aging, cause sunspots, and increase the risk of skin cancer.

Pollution: Air pollution and other environmental pollutants can damage the skin, leading to premature aging and dullness.

Diet: A healthy diet rich in fruits, vegetables, and antioxidants can nourish your skin from within, promoting a healthy glow.

Stories of Transformation

Sarah's Skin Story

For as long as Sarah could remember, her skin had been a source of frustration. Dry patches, occasional breakouts, and an overall lack of radiance made her self-conscious. She tried countless products, from drugstore staples to high-end brands, but nothing seemed to work. Worse, some products left her skin irritated and red. Feeling defeated, Sarah decided to dig deeper and understand what her skin truly needed.

Her turning point came when she attended a workshop on skin biology. For the first time, she learned about the structure and functions of the skin, from the protective barrier of the epidermis to the collagen-rich dermis. She discovered that her dry patches were caused by a compromised skin barrier and that some of the harsh products she had been using were stripping her skin of its natural oils.

With her newfound knowledge, Sarah took a more mindful approach to her skincare routine. She focused on repairing her skin barrier by using gentle cleansers, hydrating toners, and moisturizers rich in ceramides and fatty acids. She also introduced pH-balanced products to maintain her skin's natural acid mantle. Gradually, Sarah began to see remarkable changes—her dry patches disappeared, her skin became smoother, and her complexion gained a healthy glow.

Empowered by her success, Sarah continued to learn about skin biology and even started experimenting with DIY formulations tailored to her needs. For instance, she crafted a calming chamomile-infused oil cleanser to remove makeup without irritation. Sarah's journey illustrates the transformative power of understanding your skin's unique needs. Armed with the right knowledge, she not only improved her skin's health but also gained confidence and a sense of control over her skincare routine.

Key Takeaway

By understanding the intricate workings of your skin, you can truly empower yourself in your skincare journey. This knowledge provides a foundation for making informed choices about your skincare routine and creating personalized solutions that truly address your unique needs and concerns.

Think of it as unlocking the secrets of your skin. By understanding its structure, function, and how it reacts to different factors, you can identify your skin's specific needs and tailor your skincare approach accordingly. This personalized approach goes beyond simply applying products; it involves understanding your skin's unique language and communicating with it effectively.

This knowledge empowers you to:

Identify and address specific skin concerns: Whether it's dryness, oiliness, acne, or signs of aging, you can target these concerns with the most appropriate ingredients and formulations.

Choose the right products: You can make informed decisions about which commercial products are best suited for your skin type and concerns.

Create effective DIY formulations: You can confidently create your own skincare products that are tailored to your specific needs and preferences.

By taking control of your skincare knowledge, you can achieve a radiant, glowing complexion while nurturing your skin's natural health and beauty.

Crafting Your Own Skincare Solutions

Now that we understand the fundamentals of skin biology, let's roll up our sleeves and embark on the exciting journey of creating our own natural skincare products.

Just as artists use their understanding of colour theory and composition to create beautiful works of art, we can use our knowledge of skin biology to create skincare formulations that are both effective and nourishing.

This chapter will guide you through the essential steps of formulating basic skincare products. We'll explore the building blocks of skincare, including oils, butters, hydrosols, and emulsifiers, and learn how to combine them to create a variety of textures, from lightweight serums to rich, nourishing creams.

You'll also learn how to gather the necessary tools and equipment for your DIY skincare journey and discover simple recipes to get you started. We'll address important safety considerations, such as proper hygiene and patch testing, to ensure that your creations are safe and effective for your skin.

By the end of this chapter, you'll gain the confidence to experiment with different formulations, discover the joy of creating personalized skincare solutions, and embark on a rewarding journey of self-discovery and creativity.

Chapter 3: Mastering Basic Skincare Formulations

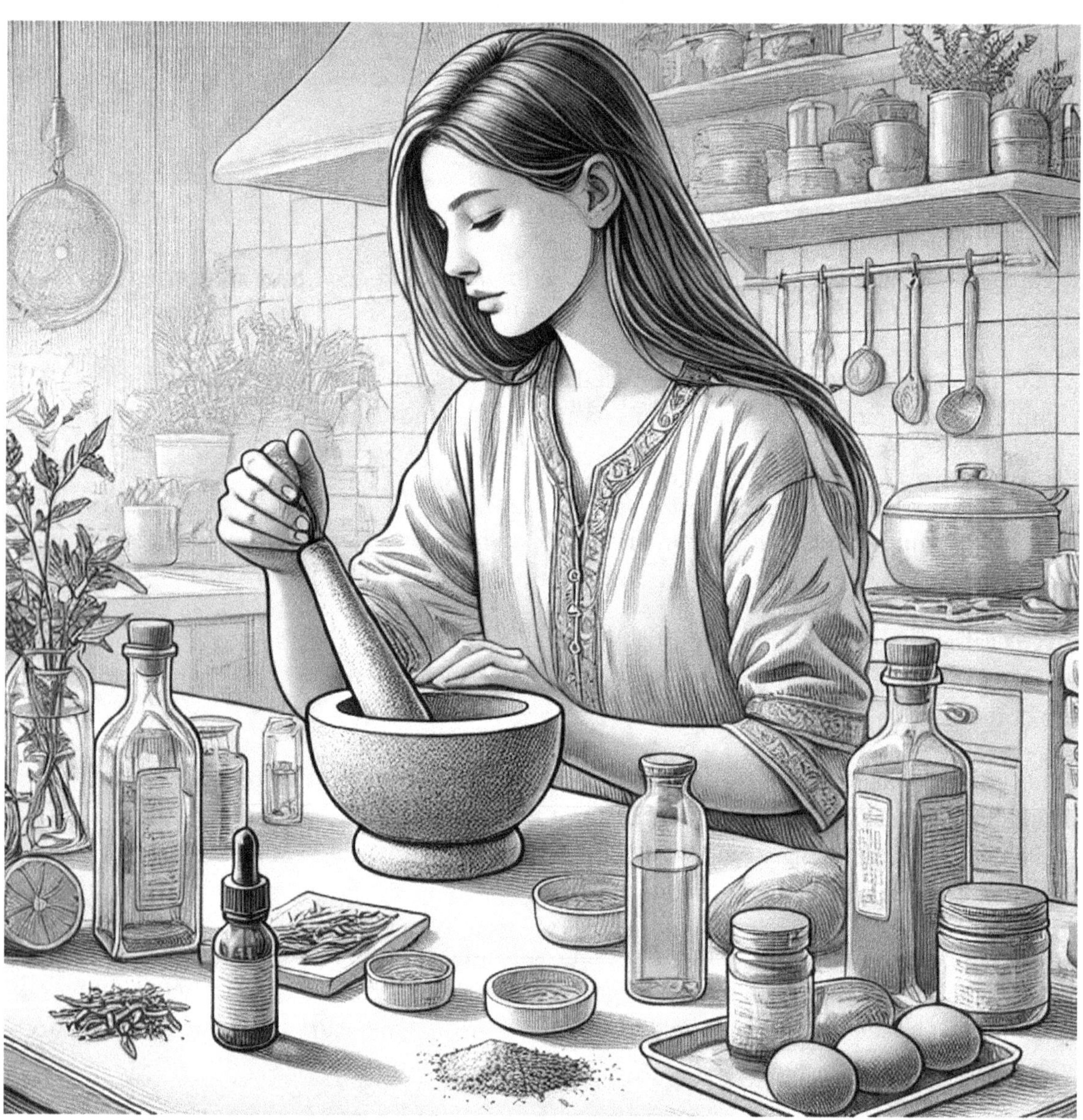

A Historical Perspective

Long before the advent of modern cosmetics, our ancestors relied on the healing properties of plants and natural ingredients to care for their skin. From Cleopatra's milk baths to the Ayurvedic traditions of India, history is replete with examples of effective natural beauty remedies. These ancient practices offer valuable insights into the power of natural ingredients and inspire us to create our own effective and sustainable skincare solutions.

Essential Formulations

Building Blocks of Skincare: Let's explore the fundamental components of skincare formulations:

Oils: Carrier oils like jojoba, argan, and sweet almond oil provide nourishment, hydration, and emollience.

Butters: Shea butter, cocoa butter, and mango butter offer deep hydration and protection, ideal for dry and sensitive skin.

Hydrosols: Floral waters like rosewater and lavender water provide gentle toning and refreshing benefits.

Emulsifiers: Ingredients like beeswax, lecithin, and vegetable glycerine help to stabilize oil and water mixtures, creating smooth and creamy emulsions.

Active Ingredients: Essential oils, botanical extracts, and vitamins offer targeted benefits, such as antioxidant protection, anti-inflammatory properties, and brightening effects.

Your DIY Skincare Toolkit: Gather the essential tools and equipment for creating your own skincare products at home:

Measuring spoons and cups: For accurate measurement of ingredients.

Bowls and spatulas: For mixing and combining ingredients.

Glass jars and bottles: For storing your finished products.

Pipettes and droppers: For precise measurement and application of essential oils and other liquid ingredients.

Mortar and pestle: For grinding herbs and creating infused oils.

Emulsions, Serums, and Balms: Let's explore the art of creating different skincare textures:

Emulsions: These lightweight, water-based formulations are ideal for oily and combination skin. They typically contain a blend of oils, water, and an emulsifier.

Serums: Highly concentrated formulations that deliver potent actives to the skin. Serums are typically lightweight and easily absorbed.

Balms: Rich, deeply hydrating formulations that are ideal for dry and sensitive skin. They often contain a high concentration of oils and butters.

Simple Recipes to Get You Started: Let's begin with some easy-to-follow recipes for popular skincare products:

Simple Moisturizing Cream: Combine shea butter, jojoba oil, and rosewater to create a nourishing and hydrating cream.

Gentle Facial Cleanser: Mix gentle cleansing oils like olive oil or coconut oil with a hydrosol like lavender water for a refreshing and effective cleanser.

Soothing Toner: Combine witch hazel, rosewater, and a few drops of tea tree oil for a refreshing and toning mist.

Safety Considerations and Troubleshooting Guides:

Safety First: Always practice good hygiene when creating skincare products. Wash your hands thoroughly before and after handling ingredients.

Patch Testing: Before applying any new product to your face, perform a patch test on a small area of skin to check for any allergic reactions.

Preservation: Learn about natural preservatives like vitamin E and grapefruit seed extract to help extend the shelf life of your creations.

Troubleshooting: Address common formulation challenges, such as separation, discoloration, and ineffective formulations. If your product separates, try gently warming it in a double boiler and stirring until it emulsifies. If your product changes colour, it may be due to oxidation. Consider adding a few drops of vitamin E oil to help prevent discoloration.

Stories of Success

From Novice to Natural Skincare Enthusiast

Emily, a creative spirit with a knack for exploring new hobbies, found herself intrigued by the idea of crafting her own skincare products. Initially, she felt overwhelmed by the sheer amount of information available—DIY recipes, ingredient lists, and safety considerations seemed daunting for someone with no prior experience. But her curiosity and desire to switch to natural, eco-friendly products drove her to take the first step.

Her journey began with a simple project: a moisturizing body butter. Armed with a few basic ingredients like shea butter, coconut oil, and essential oils, Emily followed a beginner-friendly recipe she found online. She melted the ingredients in a makeshift double boiler, stirred them together, and waited for the mixture to set. To her surprise, the result was a luxurious, creamy body butter that left her skin feeling soft and nourished.

The sense of accomplishment Emily felt was transformative. "I couldn't believe I had made this myself," she recalled. "It was such a small thing, but it felt incredibly empowering." Encouraged by her success, Emily began experimenting with other DIY projects, from herbal-infused facial oils to soothing lip balms. Each new creation deepened her appreciation for the power of natural ingredients and the artistry of formulation.

Over time, Emily developed a deeper understanding of her skin's unique needs and how to tailor products accordingly. For her dry winter skin, she crafted a lavender-scented night cream rich in cocoa butter. To combat the summer's humidity, she formulated a lightweight, aloe-based toner infused with green tea.

Emily's journey exemplifies how accessible and rewarding DIY skincare can be. What started as a simple experiment evolved into a creative outlet and a source of personal pride. Today, Emily shares her knowledge through social media, inspiring others to take their first steps into the world of DIY skincare. Her story reminds us that with curiosity, patience, and a willingness to learn, anyone can create something beautiful, effective, and uniquely their own.

Key Takeaway

With a little practice and patience, you can discover the joy and empowerment that comes with creating effective and personalized skincare solutions using natural ingredients. The process of formulating your own products is not merely about achieving a desired skin texture; it's about connecting with your skin on a deeper level and understanding its unique needs.

By experimenting with different ingredients, observing your skin's reactions, and refining your formulations, you gain a deeper understanding of your skin's needs and preferences. This hands-on experience empowers you to take control of your skincare routine and create products that truly nourish and nurture your skin.

Furthermore, the process of creating your own skincare products can be incredibly rewarding. The satisfaction of crafting something beautiful and effective with your own hands is immeasurable. It's a testament to your creativity, resourcefulness, and the power of natural ingredients.

Sourcing Sustainable Ingredients

Now that we've explored the basics of formulating skincare products, let's delve deeper into a crucial aspect of eco-friendly skincare: sourcing sustainable ingredients.

Just as we carefully consider the ingredients we use in our food; we must also be mindful of the ingredients we apply to our skin. The conventional beauty industry often relies on synthetic ingredients and unsustainable practices, contributing to environmental degradation and potential health concerns.

In this chapter, we'll explore the importance of choosing sustainable ingredients that are ethically sourced and produced with minimal environmental impact. We'll discuss the importance of supporting organic farming practices, fair trade initiatives, and choosing ingredients that are locally sourced whenever possible.

By prioritizing sustainability in our ingredient choices, we can not only nourish our skin but also contribute to a healthier planet.

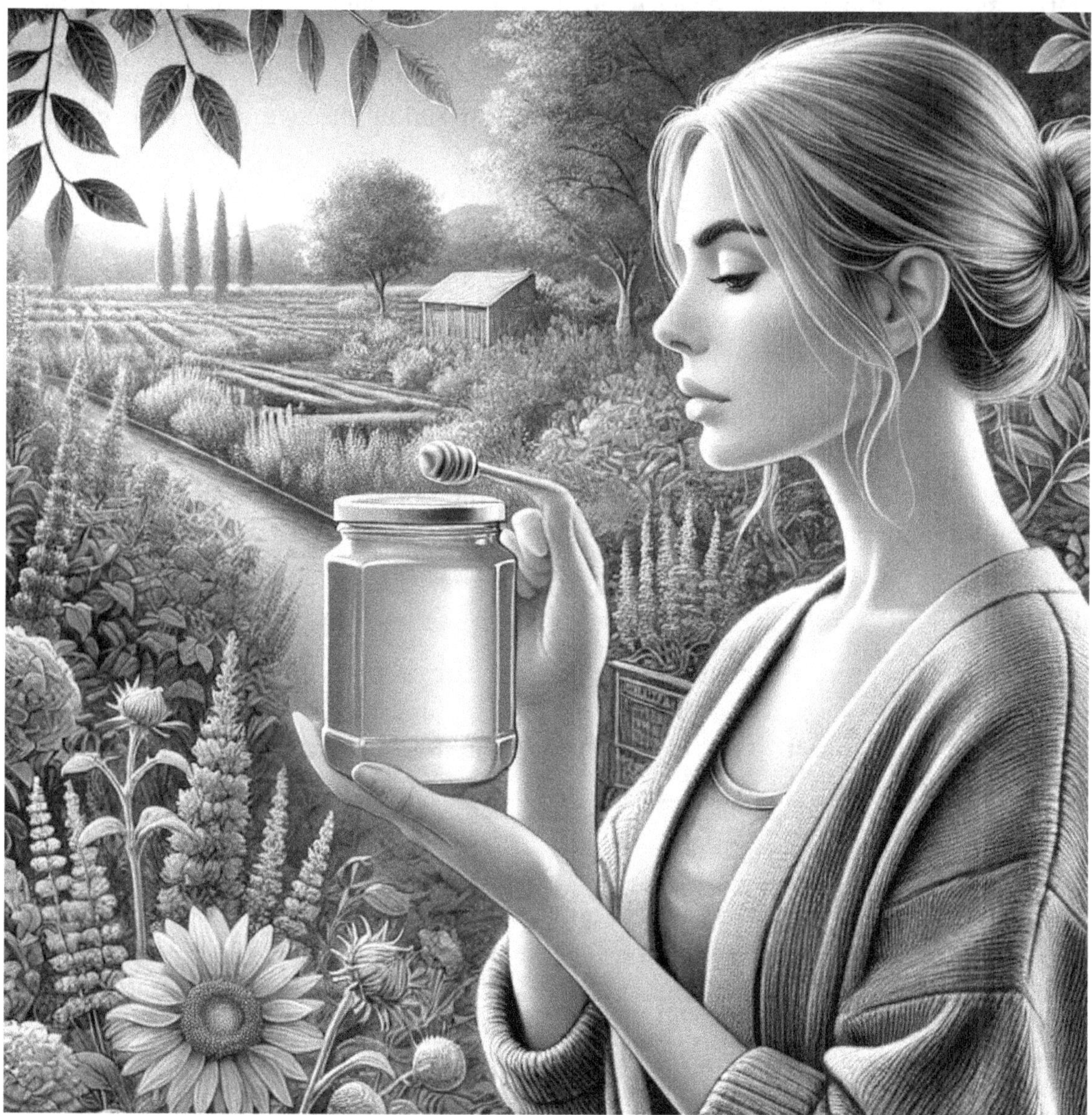

The Impact of Conventional Ingredients

The conventional beauty industry often relies on synthetic ingredients and unsustainable practices, contributing to environmental degradation and health concerns. Many conventional skincare products contain harmful chemicals like parabens, phthalates, and microplastics, which can have negative impacts on both human health and the environment.

Defining Sustainable Ingredients

What Does "Sustainable" Really Mean: Sustainable ingredients are sourced and produced in a way that minimizes environmental impact and supports social and economic equity. This includes:

Organic Certification: Look for products certified organic, indicating that the ingredients were grown without the use of synthetic pesticides, herbicides, or fertilizers.

Fair Trade Practices: Support fair trade certified ingredients, ensuring that farmers and workers receive fair wages and working conditions.

Wildcrafted with Respect: When using wildcrafted ingredients, ensure they are harvested sustainably and responsibly, without harming the environment or local ecosystems.

Minimizing Environmental Impact: Consider the environmental impact of the entire production process, from cultivation and harvesting to transportation and packaging.

Identifying Reliable Sources:

Local Farmers' Markets: Connect with local farmers and producers to source high-quality, sustainably grown ingredients.

Community Supported Agriculture (CSA) programs: Join a CSA to receive a weekly box of fresh, seasonal produce, including herbs and botanicals that can be used in your skincare.

Online Retailers: Research online retailers that specialize in selling organic, fair trade, and sustainably sourced ingredients.

Supporting Small Businesses: Choose to support small businesses that prioritize sustainability and ethical practices.

Decoding Labels: A Guide to Sustainable Certifications

Organic: Indicates that the ingredients were grown without the use of synthetic pesticides, herbicides, or fertilizers.

Fair Trade: Ensures that farmers and workers receive fair wages and working conditions.

Cruelty-Free: Indicates that the product was not tested on animals.

Vegan: Indicates that the product does not contain any animal-derived ingredients.

Minimizing Packaging Waste:

Choose bulk options: Purchase ingredients in bulk whenever possible to reduce packaging waste.

Opt for refillable containers: Invest in reusable containers and refill them with your DIY creations or purchase products from brands that offer refill options.

Choose minimal packaging: Look for products with minimal packaging and opt for recyclable or biodegradable materials.

The Power of Local: Discover the benefits of incorporating locally sourced ingredients into your skincare routine:

Reduced carbon footprint: Sourcing ingredients locally reduces transportation distances, minimizing your carbon footprint.

Supporting local economies: Supporting local farmers and producers helps to strengthen local economies and create jobs.

Access to fresh, high-quality ingredients: Locally sourced ingredients are typically fresher and more potent, offering maximum benefits for your skin.

Stories of Sustainability

A Small Business, a Big Impact

Meet Maya, a passionate entrepreneur who turned her love for natural skincare into a thriving small business with a mission to make a difference. Maya's journey began in her kitchen, where she experimented with creating simple, chemical-free skincare products for her family. As her creations gained popularity among friends and neighbors, she saw an opportunity to expand her hobby into a business that could embody her values of sustainability and community support.

From the outset, Maya was determined to prioritize locally sourced ingredients. She partnered with nearby farmers to obtain fresh herbs, organic oils, and natural waxes. By doing so, she ensured the quality of her products while supporting the local economy. Her commitment extended to her packaging choices—she used glass jars, compostable labels, and refill programs to minimize waste.

Maya's business quickly became a cornerstone of her community. Her shop not only offered sustainable skincare solutions but also served as a space for workshops on DIY skincare and environmental education. She collaborated with local artisans to create eco-friendly gift sets and donated a portion of her profits to conservation initiatives.

Her efforts didn't go unnoticed. Customers appreciated the transparency and thoughtfulness behind her brand, and word of mouth helped her business grow. Maya's story demonstrates the power of small businesses to create meaningful change. By prioritizing sustainability and community impact, she proved that conscious consumerism could inspire both individual and collective action toward a healthier planet.

A Journey of Discovery

Olivia, a dedicated hobbyist, embarked on a personal mission to incorporate sustainability into her DIY skincare creations. Initially, she relied on readily available ingredients from local stores, but as her knowledge and interest grew, she became curious about the origins of these ingredients and their environmental impact.

Determined to make more informed choices, Olivia began researching sustainable suppliers. She discovered businesses that specialized in ethically sourced and organic materials, such as cold-pressed oils and responsibly harvested botanicals. Her journey was filled with moments of discovery, like finding a cooperative that empowered rural farmers or learning about fair trade practices that ensured equitable wages for workers.

Each new supplier brought a deeper connection to her products. Olivia took the time to visit local farms and markets, meeting growers and hearing their stories. These interactions gave her a profound appreciation for the labor and care involved in producing high-quality, sustainable ingredients. The relationships she built with suppliers became a source of inspiration, enriching her understanding of sustainability and ethical business practices.

As Olivia integrated these ingredients into her skincare formulations, she felt a renewed sense of purpose. She began sharing her discoveries with friends and fellow hobbyists, encouraging them to support ethical businesses and explore the joys of sustainable living. Olivia's journey highlights the importance of research and the rewarding experience of connecting with like-minded individuals who share a commitment to protecting the planet.

Her story serves as a reminder that even small steps, like choosing sustainable suppliers, can lead to profound personal growth and contribute to a larger movement for ethical and environmentally friendly practices.

Key Takeaway

By consciously choosing sustainable ingredients, we are not merely selecting products for our skincare routines; we are making a conscious decision to support a more ethical and sustainable beauty industry.

Nourishing our Skin and the Planet: When we choose organic, fair trade, and locally sourced ingredients, we are not only nourishing our skin but also supporting sustainable agricultural practices, fair labour conditions, and the health of our planet.

Reducing our Environmental Impact: By prioritizing sustainable ingredients, we minimize our contribution to environmental issues such as deforestation, soil erosion, and water pollution.

Supporting Ethical Sourcing: When we choose products that support fair trade practices, we ensure that farmers and workers receive fair wages and working conditions, promoting social and economic equity.

Empowering Change: By making conscious choices as consumers, we send a powerful message to the beauty industry, encouraging them to prioritize sustainability and ethical practices.

Supporting ethical sourcing practices, minimizing packaging waste, and choosing locally sourced ingredients are all steps towards a more sustainable and equitable beauty industry.

By making these conscious choices, we can contribute to a healthier planet for ourselves and future generations.

Personalizing Your Skincare Routine

Now that we've explored the importance of sustainable ingredients, let's delve into the art of personalizing your skincare routine to achieve optimal results.

Just as every snowflake is unique, so is your skin. What works wonders for your friend might not be the best fit for you. The key to achieving radiant skin lies in creating a personalized skincare routine that addresses your specific needs and preferences.

This chapter will guide you through the process of tailoring your skincare routine to your individual skin type, concerns, and lifestyle. We'll explore how to adjust your formulations to address specific needs, such as dryness, oiliness, acne, and sensitivity. You'll learn how to customize the texture and scent of your products to create a truly enjoyable skincare experience.

Furthermore, we'll discuss the importance of adapting your skincare routine to seasonal changes and explore strategies for tracking your skin's progress and adjusting as needed. By embracing the art of experimentation and tailoring your routine to your unique needs, you can unlock your skin's full potential and achieve a truly radiant complexion.

Chapter 5: Customizing Your Skincare Routine

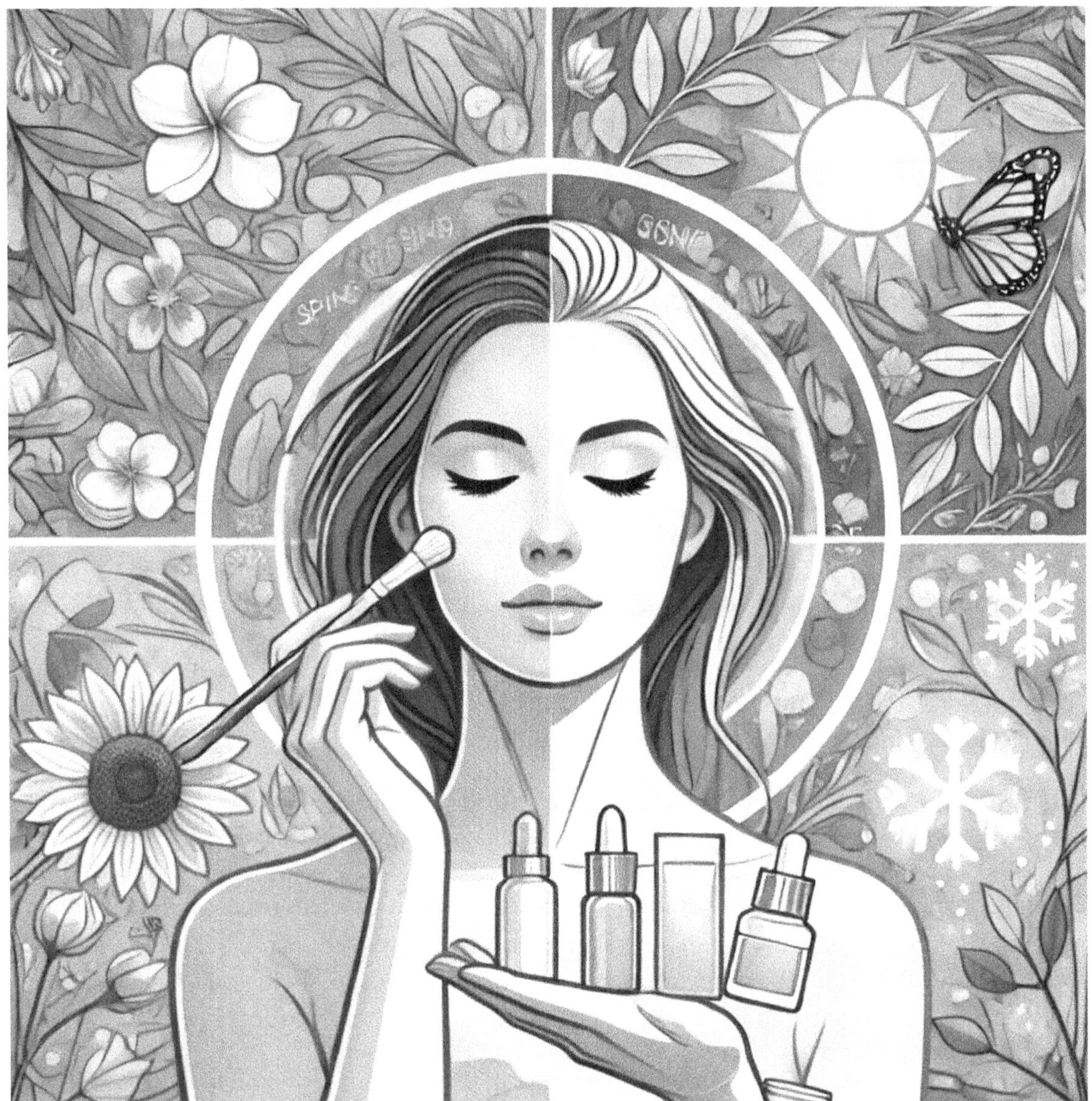

Oily skin: Incorporate ingredients like clay, tea tree oil, and witch hazel to help absorb excess oil and minimize breakouts.

Dry skin: Focus on hydrating ingredients like shea butter, coconut oil, and hyaluronic acid to replenish moisture and soothe dryness.

Sensitive skin: Choose gentle, non-irritating ingredients like aloe vera, chamomile, and calendula to soothe and calm the skin.

Acne-prone skin: Incorporate ingredients like tea tree oil, witch hazel, and niacinamide to help regulate oil production and prevent breakouts.

Texture and Scent Preferences: Explore ways to customize the texture and scent of your products to create a truly enjoyable skincare experience:

Experiment with different oils: Choose oils with textures that you enjoy, such as lightweight jojoba oil or rich shea butter.

Incorporate essential oils: Add a few drops of your favourite essential oils to your formulations to create a pleasant aroma. Lavender oil is known for its calming properties, while rose oil has a romantic and uplifting scent.

Consider your personal preferences: If you prefer lightweight, quickly absorbing products, opt for serums and lotions. If you enjoy a richer, more luxurious feel, choose creams and balms.

Seasonal Shifts: Discover how to adapt your skincare routine to seasonal changes:

Summer: Protect your skin from the sun with a broad-spectrum sunscreen and incorporate lightweight, hydrating products to combat the effects of heat and humidity.

Winter: Deeply hydrate your skin with rich creams and oils to combat dryness and protect it from harsh winter weather.

Spring: Transition to lighter formulations and incorporate exfoliating ingredients to gently remove dead skin cells and reveal a brighter complexion.

Fall: Prepare your skin for the colder months by increasing hydration and incorporating antioxidant-rich ingredients to protect against environmental damage.

Tracking Progress and Adjusting: Keep a skincare journal to track your progress and adjust your routine as needed. Note down any changes in your skin's condition, the products you are using, and any noticeable improvements or concerns. This will help you identify what works best for your skin and make informed decisions about your skincare routine.

The Art of Experimentation: Embrace the process of experimentation and discover the joy of creating unique skincare blends that truly nourish your skin. Don't be afraid to try new ingredients and formulations and have fun with the process!

Stories of Personalization

A Skin Journey, A Personal Triumph

Claire had always struggled with her skin. Oily in some areas and dry in others, her combination skin presented challenges that even professional consultations couldn't fully resolve. She often found herself frustrated as she tried products marketed as "universal solutions," only to end up with more clogged pores or patchy dryness.

One day, after a particularly severe breakout, Claire decided to take matters into her own hands. She began researching skincare and discovered the importance of tailoring a routine to her unique skin type and concerns. Armed with newfound knowledge, she set out to experiment and develop a regimen that would work specifically for her.

Claire started by identifying her skin's needs. For her oily T-zone, she incorporated lightweight, mattifying products like a niacinamide serum and a clay-based mask to control excess sebum. For her dry cheeks, she added deeply hydrating products, including rosehip oil and a ceramide-rich moisturizer. She also introduced gentle exfoliation to address dullness, using a lactic acid serum twice a week.

The results were transformative. Over time, Claire's skin became balanced, with fewer breakouts and a healthy, natural glow. Her newfound confidence extended beyond her physical appearance—she felt empowered by her ability to understand and meet her skin's needs. "The key was listening to my skin," Claire shared. "Once I stopped chasing trends and started focusing on what worked for me, everything changed."

Claire now advocates for the importance of a personalized skincare approach, encouraging others to observe their skin's reactions and adjust their routines accordingly. Her journey demonstrates that taking the time to understand your skin can lead to remarkable results and a deeper sense of self-care.

Cultural Adaptations - A Global Perspective

Skincare practices have always been influenced by the environments and cultural traditions of different regions. These adaptations provide valuable lessons for creating routines that suit diverse climates and skin needs.

In tropical climates with high humidity, such as Southeast Asia, lighter, water-based formulations are popular. People often use cooling gels, refreshing mists, and lightweight moisturizers that quickly absorb into the skin. Ingredients like cucumber, aloe vera, and green tea are common, offering hydration without clogging pores.

Conversely, in arid and desert regions like North Africa, the focus is on deep hydration and protection against moisture loss. Rich oils like argan and shea butter are staples, used to nourish the skin and shield it from harsh environmental conditions. These ingredients not only provide hydration but also form a protective barrier to lock in moisture.

In colder climates, such as Scandinavia, skincare routines emphasize protection against windburn and extreme dryness. Thick creams infused with fatty acids and humectants like glycerin are common. Additionally, cultural practices such as sauna therapy are integrated into skincare, helping to detoxify and rejuvenate the skin.

Even within similar climates, cultural practices can vary widely. For instance, in Japan, a meticulous, multi-step routine focuses on layering lightweight, hydrating products to achieve a radiant, dewy complexion. Meanwhile, in the Mediterranean, skincare often incorporates antioxidant-rich ingredients like olive oil and pomegranate, reflecting the region's agricultural abundance.

These cultural adaptations highlight the universal goal of skincare—nurturing the skin in harmony with the environment. By understanding these traditions, modern skincare enthusiasts can draw inspiration to create routines that align with both their unique skin needs and the climate they live in. This global perspective reminds us that skincare is not one-size-fits-all; it's a deeply personal practice shaped by heritage, environment, and individual preferences.

Key Takeaway

By understanding your skin's unique needs and preferences, you can create a personalized skincare routine that is both effective and enjoyable. This journey of self-discovery is a deeply personal one, and there is no one-size-fits-all approach.

Embrace Your Individuality: Every individual has unique skin and unique needs. What works for one person may not work for another. By embracing the individuality of your skin and carefully observing its reactions, you can develop a customized routine that truly nourishes and protects.

The Power of Observation: Pay close attention to how your skin reacts to different products and environmental factors. This will help you identify your skin's unique needs and preferences, such as sensitivity to certain ingredients, reactions to weather changes, and the impact of your diet.

Embrace the Process: The journey of discovering the perfect skincare regimen is an ongoing process of experimentation and refinement. Be patient with yourself and enjoy the process of learning and discovering what works best for your skin.

Celebrate Small Victories: Acknowledge and celebrate small successes along the way, such as identifying a new ingredient that works wonders for your skin or creating a formulation that you absolutely love.

This journey is about more than just achieving clear skin; it's about developing a deeper understanding of yourself and your relationship with your skin. By embracing the process of self-discovery and experimentation, you can create a skincare routine that is not only effective but also enjoyable and empowering.

From Passion to Profit

For some, the passion for DIY skincare may evolve into a desire to share their creations with the world. Perhaps you've developed a signature blend that consistently delivers amazing results, or maybe you've discovered a unique and effective way to incorporate sustainable practices into your skincare routine.

This chapter will explore the exciting possibility of turning your passion for eco-friendly skincare into a thriving business. We'll delve into the essential steps involved in starting a skincare business, from developing a business plan to building a strong brand identity and navigating the complexities of the market.

Whether you dream of launching a small, handcrafted skincare line or building a larger, more impactful brand, this chapter will provide you with the information and inspiration you need to turn your passion into a successful and fulfilling business venture.

Chapter 6: Launching Your Skincare Business

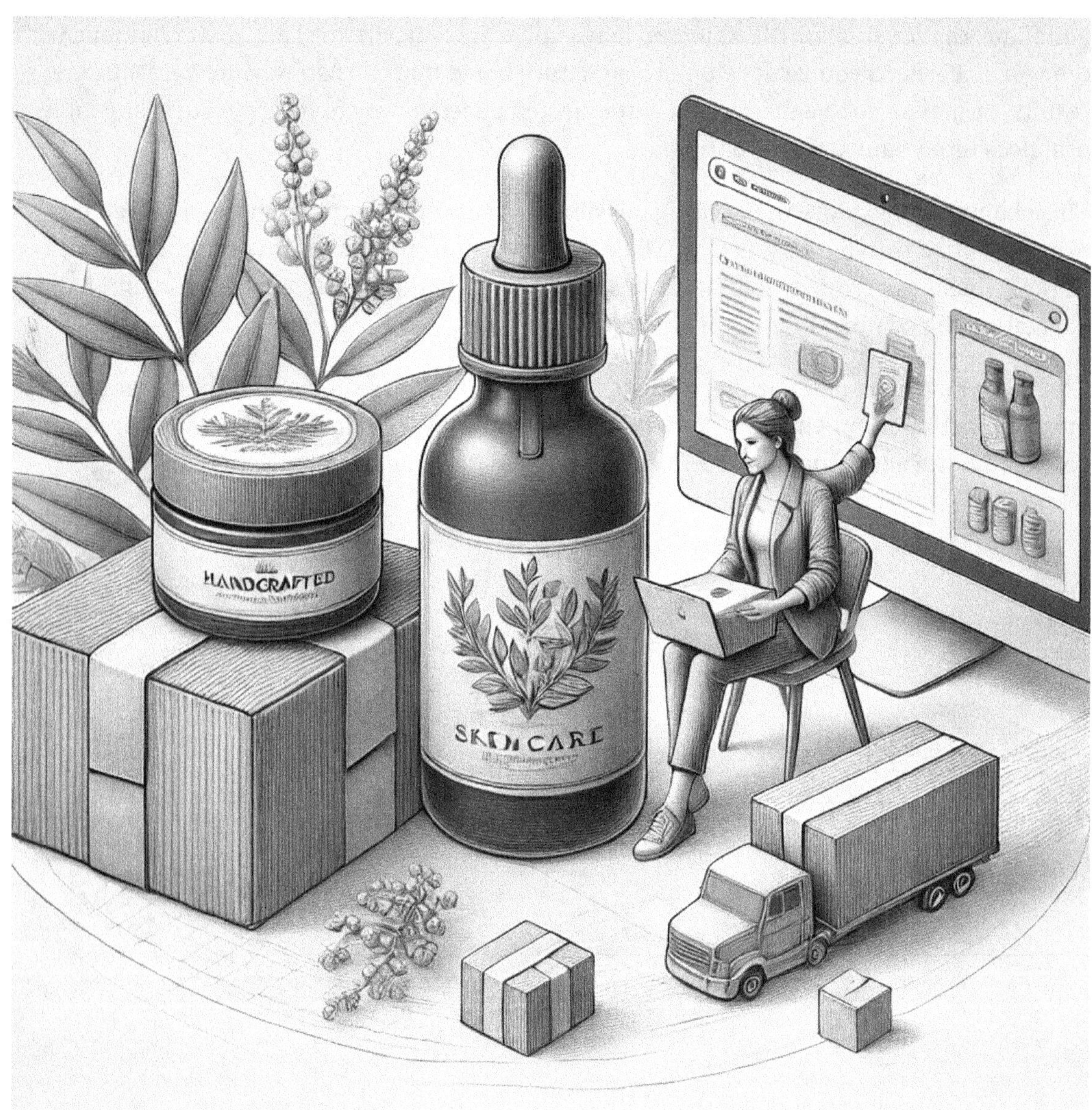

Turning Your Passion into a Profit

Transforming your passion for eco-friendly skincare into a successful business requires careful planning, creativity, and a deep understanding of the market.

The Foundations of a Skincare Business:

Develop a Business Plan: Outline your business goals, target market, and financial projections.

Choose a Business Structure: Determine the legal structure of your business, such as a sole proprietorship, partnership, or LLC.

Obtain Necessary Licenses and Permits: Research and obtain any necessary licenses and permits required to operate your business in your area.

Secure Funding: Explore funding options, such as personal savings, loans, or seeking investors.

Understanding Your Market:

Identify Your Target Audience: Define your ideal customer, considering their demographics, interests, and skincare needs.

Analyse Market Trends: Research current trends in the skincare industry, including consumer preferences, emerging ingredients, and innovative packaging.

Competitive Analysis: Analyse your competition, identifying their strengths and weaknesses and identifying opportunities to differentiate your brand.

Branding and Marketing:

Develop a Strong Brand Identity: Create a compelling brand story and visual identity that resonates with your target audience.

Create High-Quality Marketing Materials: Develop professional-looking website, social media content, and product packaging.

Explore Sustainable Marketing Strategies: Utilize environmentally friendly marketing practices, such as email marketing, social media marketing, and influencer collaborations.

Legal and Ethical Considerations:

Product Labelling: Ensure that your product labels comply with all relevant regulations, including ingredient lists, warnings, and safety information.

Safety Testing: Conduct thorough safety testing on your products to ensure they are safe for use.

Ethical Sourcing and Manufacturing: Prioritize ethical sourcing and manufacturing practices, ensuring fair wages and safe working conditions for all employees.

Pricing and Scaling Your Business:

Determine Competitive Pricing: Research competitor pricing and determine a competitive price point for your products.

Explore Pricing Strategies: Consider offering tiered pricing options, subscription services, or bundle deals.

Develop a Scalability Plan: Plan for future growth and scalability, considering factors such as increased production capacity and expanding your product line.

Stories of Entrepreneurship

From Kitchen to Commerce

Follow the inspiring journey of Elara, a passionate home cook who discovered a love for natural skincare after years of struggling with sensitive skin. Frustrated by the lack of effective and natural options, she began experimenting in her kitchen, crafting simple yet effective remedies for herself.

Elara's friends and family quickly took notice of her glowing skin and began requesting her creations. Recognizing the potential, Elara decided to turn her passion into a business. She started small, selling her handcrafted soaps and balms at local farmers' markets. Through word-of-mouth and social media, her business began to grow. Elara remained committed to using only the highest quality, ethically sourced ingredients, and minimizing her environmental impact. Today, her small, homegrown business has blossomed into a thriving brand, inspiring others to pursue their own entrepreneurial dreams and embrace sustainable living.

Sustainability in Action

Explore the story of "Terra & Tide," a small skincare brand founded by a group of friends with a shared passion for sustainability. From the very beginning, Terra & Tide prioritized ethical sourcing, using organic, fair-trade ingredients whenever possible. They chose to minimize packaging waste by using recyclable glass bottles and minimal, compostable inserts.

Furthermore, Terra & Tide actively supports environmental conservation efforts by partnering with local organizations and donating a portion of their profits to environmental causes. Their commitment to sustainability has not only resonated with their customers but has also inspired other businesses in the beauty industry to embrace more eco-conscious practices.

These stories highlight the power of passion, perseverance, and a commitment to sustainability. They demonstrate that building a successful and impactful business is not just about creating a profit; it's about creating a positive impact on the world and inspiring others to embrace a more sustainable way of life.

Key Takeaway

With careful planning, dedication, and a commitment to sustainability, turning your passion for eco-friendly skincare into a successful business is an achievable and rewarding endeavour.

More Than Just Profit: Building a successful business goes beyond simply generating revenue. It's about creating a positive impact on the world, aligning your business practices with your values, and making a meaningful contribution to society.

Prioritizing Ethical Practices: This involves prioritizing ethical sourcing, fair labour practices, and minimizing your environmental impact at every stage of the business, from production and distribution to customer service.

Building a Brand with Purpose: By building a strong brand that embodies your values and resonates with conscious consumers, you can attract loyal customers who share your commitment to sustainability.

Creating a Positive Impact: By prioritizing ethical practices and giving back to the community, you can create a business that not only generates revenue but also makes a positive contribution to society and the environment.

By building a strong brand, prioritizing ethical practices, and providing exceptional customer service, you can create a thriving business that aligns with your values and makes a positive impact on the world.

Beyond Products: Sustainable Business Practices

Building a successful eco-friendly skincare business extends beyond creating exceptional products. It requires a deep-seated commitment to sustainability in all aspects of operations.

A Holistic Approach: Sustainability should be woven into the fabric of your entire business, from sourcing ingredients and manufacturing processes to packaging, shipping, and customer engagement.

Minimizing Environmental Impact:

Reduce, Reuse, recycle: Implement strategies to minimize waste throughout your operations, such as reducing packaging, reusing materials, and implementing robust recycling programs.

Conserve Resources: Minimize energy consumption by utilizing energy-efficient equipment and exploring renewable energy sources.

Minimize Water Usage: Implement water-efficient practices in your production and manufacturing processes.

Social Responsibility:

Fair Labor Practices: Ensure fair wages, safe working conditions, and ethical treatment for all employees throughout your supply chain.

Supporting Local Communities: Source ingredients locally whenever possible, supporting local economies and reducing transportation distances.

Giving Back: Consider giving back to the community through charitable donations, employee volunteer programs, or by supporting local environmental initiatives.

By integrating sustainability into every aspect of your business, you can create a truly ethical and impactful brand that aligns with the values of conscious consumers and contributes to a more sustainable future.

Chapter 7: Integrating Eco-Friendly Practices in Business

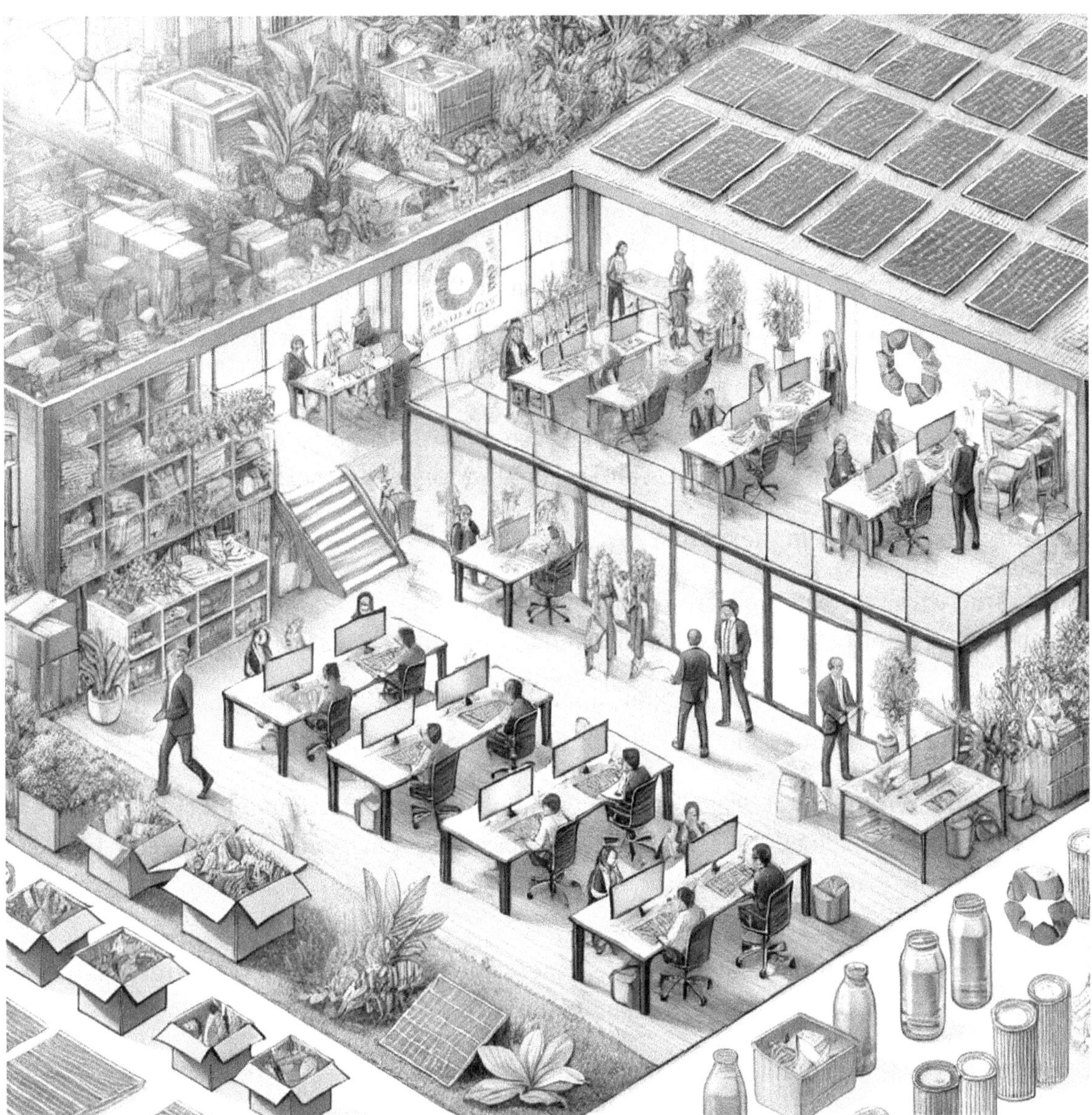

The Ethical Imperative

As businesses, we have a responsibility to minimize our environmental impact and contribute to a more sustainable future. Integrating eco-friendly practices into all aspects of your business operations is not only ethical but also enhances brand credibility and attracts conscious consumers.

Sustainable Operations:

Minimize Energy Consumption: Implement energy-efficient lighting, utilize renewable energy sources, and encourage employees to conserve energy.

Reduce Waste: Implement recycling and composting programs, minimize paper waste through digital communication, and explore options for reducing water consumption.

Invest in Green Technology: Explore the use of green technology, such as solar panels and rainwater harvesting systems, to reduce your environmental impact.

Eco-Friendly Packaging and Shipping:

Choose Sustainable Packaging: Opt for recyclable, biodegradable, or compostable packaging materials, such as glass jars, cardboard boxes, and recycled paper.

Minimize Packaging: Reduce the amount of packaging used by eliminating unnecessary components and optimizing package size.

Explore Sustainable Shipping Options: Choose eco-friendly shipping methods, such as carbon-neutral shipping or using local and regional shipping partners.

Building Sustainable Partnerships:

Collaborate with Ethical Suppliers: Partner with suppliers who share your commitment to sustainability, prioritizing ethical sourcing and fair labour practices.

Support Local Communities: Source ingredients and materials locally whenever possible, supporting local economies and reducing transportation distances.

Engage with Environmental Organizations: Collaborate with environmental organizations to support conservation efforts and raise awareness about environmental issues.

Engaging Your Customers:

Educate Your Customers: Educate your customers about your sustainability efforts and encourage them to participate in eco-friendly initiatives.

Offer Incentives for Sustainable Choices: Encourage customers to choose sustainable shipping options or return empty containers for refilling.

Collect Customer Feedback: Gather customer feedback on your sustainability efforts and use it to continuously improve your practices.

Stories of Impact

A Brand That Makes a Difference

"Terra & Tide," a trailblazing skincare brand, has emerged as a shining example of sustainability in the beauty industry. Founded by a group of friends united by their passion for the environment, the brand was born from a shared dream: to create high-quality, effective skincare products that minimize harm to the planet. From its inception, Terra & Tide has been committed to ethical sourcing, eco-conscious practices, and giving back to the community.

Sourcing with Integrity

Terra & Tide's approach to sourcing sets it apart. The brand partners with local farmers to procure organic, sustainably grown ingredients. By prioritizing local suppliers, they not only reduce their carbon footprint but also support small-scale agricultural communities. Ingredients like lavender, calendula, and chamomile are harvested responsibly, ensuring the preservation of biodiversity and the health of the soil.

Plastic-Free Packaging

Determined to address the issue of plastic pollution, Terra & Tide made a bold commitment: all packaging is entirely plastic-free. Their products are housed in recyclable glass jars and bottles, while labels and shipping materials are made from compostable paper and plant-based inks. The brand also offers a refill program, encouraging customers to return empty containers for reuse, further reducing waste.

Giving Back to Nature

Terra & Tide's commitment to sustainability extends beyond its products. A significant portion of their profits is donated to environmental organizations focused on ocean conservation and reforestation. These contributions help combat deforestation, restore marine ecosystems, and raise awareness about the urgent need for environmental stewardship.

Inspiring Change

Terra & Tide's efforts have not gone unnoticed. The brand has become a beacon of inspiration for consumers and businesses alike, proving that profitability and sustainability can coexist. Their success encourages other companies to adopt ethical and eco-friendly practices, contributing to a ripple effect across the beauty industry.

The Power of Collective Action

The beauty industry faces daunting environmental challenges, from the mountains of plastic waste it generates to the unsustainable harvesting of natural resources. Recognizing that these issues are too large for any single entity to tackle alone, a group of leading beauty brands came together to form the Sustainable Beauty Alliance.

Uniting for a Common Goal

The Sustainable Beauty Alliance represents a groundbreaking shift in the industry. Competitors have set aside rivalry to collaborate on solutions to shared challenges. The alliance focuses on creating industry-wide standards for sustainability, ensuring that all brands—large and small—can contribute to a healthier planet.

Driving Innovation

By pooling resources and expertise, alliance members have pioneered innovations such as biodegradable packaging, waterless formulations, and carbon-neutral shipping methods. These advancements not only reduce the environmental footprint of individual brands but also set new benchmarks for the entire industry.

Advocacy and Awareness

The alliance plays a crucial role in advocating for policy changes that support sustainability. From lobbying for bans on harmful chemicals to promoting incentives for zero-waste practices, they actively engage with policymakers to drive systemic change. At the same time, they educate consumers about the environmental impact of their choices, empowering them to demand better practices from the brands they support.

Inspiring Other Industries

The impact of the Sustainable Beauty Alliance extends beyond the beauty sector. Their success has inspired similar collaborations in industries such as fashion, food, and technology, proving that collective action is a powerful tool for addressing global environmental challenges.

Key Takeaway

By integrating eco-friendly practices into all aspects of your business operations, you can create a truly sustainable and ethical brand that aligns with the values of conscious consumers. Building a sustainable business is not just about creating exceptional products; it's about operating with integrity and making a positive impact on the world.

Beyond Profit: True success lies in creating a business that not only generates revenue but also contributes to a healthier planet and a more equitable society.

A Holistic Approach: Sustainability should be woven into the very fabric of your business, from sourcing and production to distribution and customer engagement.

A Commitment to Ethical Practices: This includes prioritizing ethical sourcing, fair labor practices, and minimizing environmental impact at every stage of the business lifecycle.

Building a Brand with Purpose: By aligning your business with your values and prioritizing sustainability, you can build a strong brand that resonates with conscious consumers who are seeking authentic and ethical brands.

A Global Impact

Our individual skincare choices have a profound impact on the planet. Let's explore how eco-friendly skincare practices intersect with global sustainability efforts.

This chapter will delve into the interconnectedness of our individual actions and the global challenges facing our planet. We'll explore how the beauty industry contributes to environmental issues, such as plastic pollution, water scarcity, and deforestation.

Furthermore, we'll discuss the power of conscious consumerism and how our individual choices can make a significant difference. By choosing sustainable products, supporting ethical brands, and embracing zero-waste practices, we can contribute to a more sustainable and equitable future for all.

This chapter will also explore the importance of collective action and the role of cross-industry collaboration in driving positive change within the beauty industry. By working together, businesses, consumers, and environmental organizations can create a more sustainable and beautiful future for generations to come.

Chapter 8: The Environmental Impact of Skincare Choices

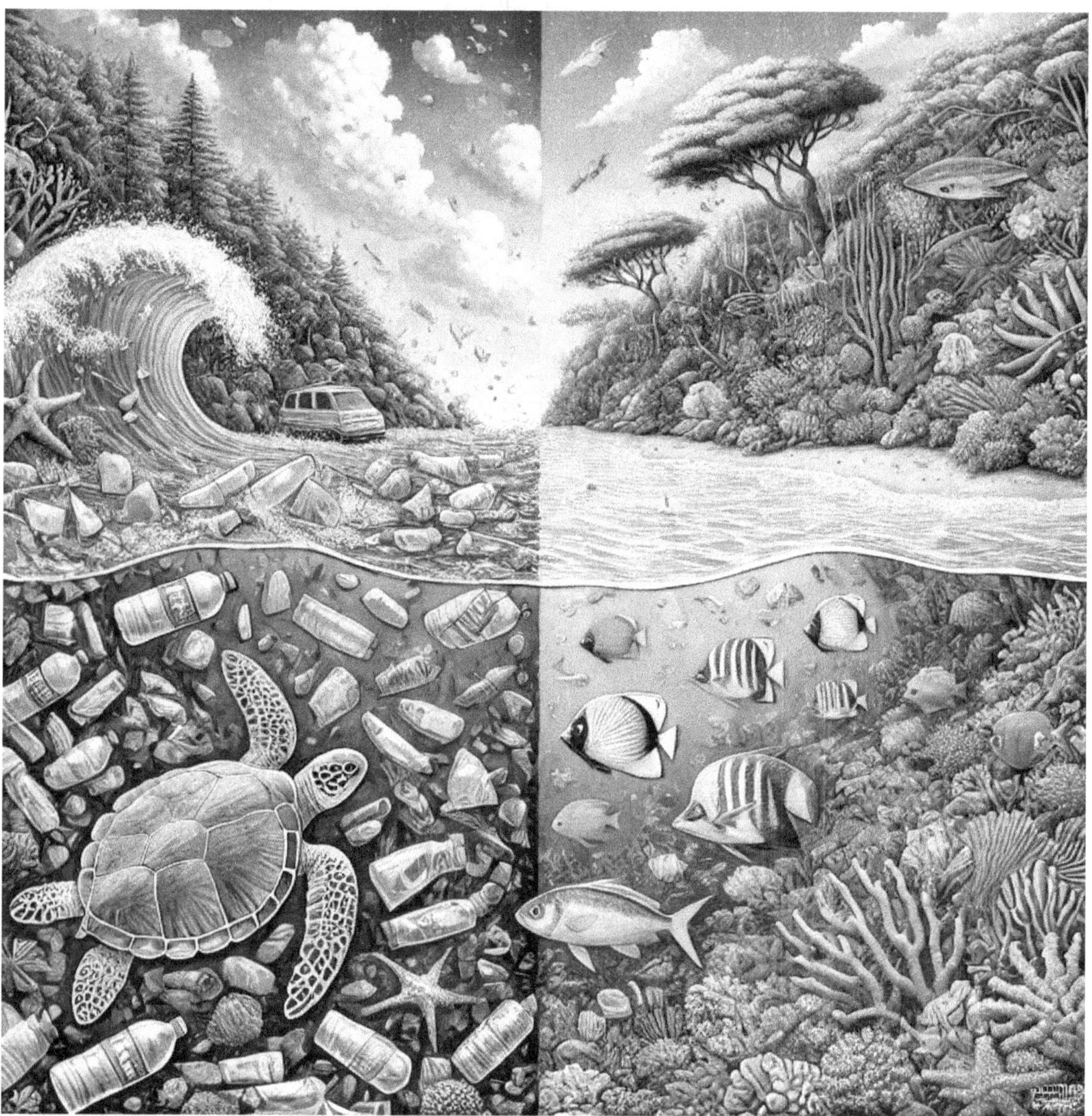

The Beauty Industry's Footprint

The conventional beauty industry contributes significantly to environmental degradation, from plastic pollution to the depletion of natural resources.

The Beauty Industry's Environmental Footprint:

Plastic Pollution: The excessive use of plastic packaging in the beauty industry contributes significantly to plastic pollution, harming marine life and polluting our oceans.

Water Consumption: The production of many beauty products requires significant amounts of water, contributing to water scarcity in some regions.

Deforestation: The cultivation of certain ingredients, such as palm oil, can contribute to deforestation and habitat loss.

Chemical Pollution: The release of harmful chemicals into the environment can contaminate water sources and harm wildlife.

The Power of Sustainable Choices:

Reduce, Reuse, recycle: Minimize waste by choosing products with minimal packaging, refilling containers, and recycling whenever possible.

Choose Products with Sustainable Packaging: Opt for products with recyclable or biodegradable packaging, such as glass jars, cardboard boxes, and paper-based materials.

Support Brands with Sustainable Practices: Choose to support brands that prioritize sustainability in all aspects of their operations, from sourcing ingredients to minimizing their environmental impact.

Embracing Zero-Waste Living: Explore strategies for minimizing waste in all areas of your life:

Reduce plastic consumption: Avoid single-use plastics and choose reusable alternatives, such as water bottles, shopping bags, and food containers.

Compost organic waste: Compost food scraps, yard waste, and other organic materials to create nutrient-rich soil.

Minimize energy consumption: Reduce your energy consumption by using energy-efficient appliances, unplugging electronics when not in use, and utilizing natural light whenever possible.

Collective Impact: How Individual Choices Matter:

The Butterfly Effect: Understand how your individual choices, such as choosing a product with minimal packaging or supporting a sustainable brand, can have a ripple effect, inspiring others to make conscious choices.

Advocacy and Education: Educate yourself and others about the environmental impact of the beauty industry and advocate for change within the industry and within your own community.

The Future of Sustainable Beauty:

Innovation and Circularity: Explore the future of the beauty industry, envisioning a future where innovation drives circularity, with products designed for reuse and recycling, and minimal waste generated throughout the entire product lifecycle.

Regenerative Practices: Support brands that prioritize regenerative practices, such as supporting local communities, restoring ecosystems, and minimizing their environmental impact.

Stories of Inspiration

A Personal Journey of Transformation

Meet Alex, a young professional who began her eco-friendly skincare journey with a simple desire to address her persistent skin issues. Frustrated by products loaded with synthetic chemicals and excessive packaging, Alex decided to explore DIY skincare and natural alternatives. She started small, crafting a basic aloe vera and chamomile toner, and was amazed at how well it soothed her sensitive skin.

This small step opened the door to a profound lifestyle transformation. As Alex delved deeper into sustainable skincare, she became more aware of her overall consumption habits. She realized the impact of single-use plastics and began seeking ways to reduce waste in her daily life. Refillable containers replaced disposable bottles, reusable cloths replaced single-use wipes, and composting became a routine practice.

Inspired by the idea of supporting local economies, Alex started sourcing her skincare ingredients from nearby farmers' markets. She was thrilled to discover high-quality organic oils and botanicals grown sustainably in her region. Her interactions with local farmers deepened her appreciation for the effort and care that went into producing these ingredients.

Alex's eco-conscious choices gradually extended beyond skincare. She switched to locally grown produce, minimized fast fashion purchases, and even began advocating for zero-waste practices in her workplace. Her journey is a powerful testament to the interconnectedness of our choices—the decision to embrace eco-friendly skincare became the catalyst for broader lifestyle changes that benefited both her community and the planet.

An Industry Shift: Towards a Sustainable Future

The beauty industry, once criticized for its heavy reliance on plastic packaging and environmentally harmful practices, is now undergoing a transformative shift toward sustainability. This movement is being driven by visionary businesses and individuals who recognize the urgency of adopting eco-friendly practices.

Leading by Example

Brands like "Terra & Tide" and others have set new benchmarks for the industry. They prioritize biodegradable packaging, ethically sourced ingredients, and carbon-neutral operations. These pioneers not only meet consumer demand for greener products but also challenge traditional business models to prove that sustainability and profitability can coexist.

Innovative Approaches

Start-ups and established brands alike are exploring innovative solutions to reduce their environmental impact. Waterless beauty products, for example, minimize water usage and packaging requirements while delivering concentrated formulas that are more efficient and environmentally friendly. Additionally, refillable packaging systems are gaining traction, allowing consumers to purchase products without contributing to landfill waste.

Empowering Consumers

The industry's shift is bolstered by consumer education initiatives that encourage mindful purchasing. Campaigns highlighting the environmental impact of beauty products—such as the lifecycle of plastic packaging or the sourcing of rare ingredients—empower consumers to make informed decisions and support brands aligned with their values.

Collaboration for Change

The formation of alliances like the Sustainable Beauty Alliance underscores the importance of collaboration in driving systemic change. By uniting competitors to share resources, establish sustainability standards, and advocate for policy changes, the alliance amplifies the industry's collective impact and sets a precedent for other sectors.

A Hopeful Future

These stories of innovation and collaboration provide hope for a future where sustainability is not an option but the cornerstone of the beauty industry. As more businesses embrace ethical practices and consumers demand greater accountability, the industry is poised to become a model for environmental stewardship.

The shift towards sustainability is a powerful reminder that individual actions, collective efforts, and innovative thinking can create meaningful change. Together, businesses and consumers have the potential to transform the beauty industry into a force for good—one that enhances beauty while preserving the planet.

Key Takeaway

By making conscious choices in our skincare routines and embracing sustainable living practices, we can contribute to a healthier planet for ourselves and future generations. Our individual actions, when combined with collective efforts, can create a powerful movement towards a more sustainable and equitable future for all.

This is more than just a personal endeavour; it's about recognizing our interconnectedness with the planet and taking responsibility for our impact.

Beyond Individual Action: While individual choices are crucial, it's equally important to recognize the power of collective action. By supporting sustainable brands, advocating for change within the beauty industry, and engaging in community efforts, we can amplify our impact and create a ripple effect that extends far beyond our individual actions.

A Shared Responsibility: We all share a responsibility to protect our planet and ensure a healthy and sustainable future for generations to come. By embracing eco-conscious practices in our daily lives, including our skincare routines, we contribute to a global movement towards a more sustainable and equitable world.

The Science of Natural Ingredients

Now that we understand the importance of sustainable practices, let's delve deeper into the science behind the natural ingredients that nourish and protect our skin.

For centuries, people have relied on the healing properties of plants and natural ingredients to care for their skin. Traditional medicine systems, such as Ayurveda and Traditional Chinese Medicine, have long recognized the therapeutic benefits of botanicals.

In this chapter, we'll explore the science behind these powerful natural ingredients, from their unique chemical compositions to their mechanisms of action on the skin. We'll delve into the rich history of herbal remedies and explore the scientific evidence supporting the efficacy of various botanicals in addressing different skin concerns.

By understanding the science behind natural ingredients, we can harness their power to create effective and nourishing skincare solutions while minimizing our environmental impact.

Chapter 9: Understanding Natural Ingredients

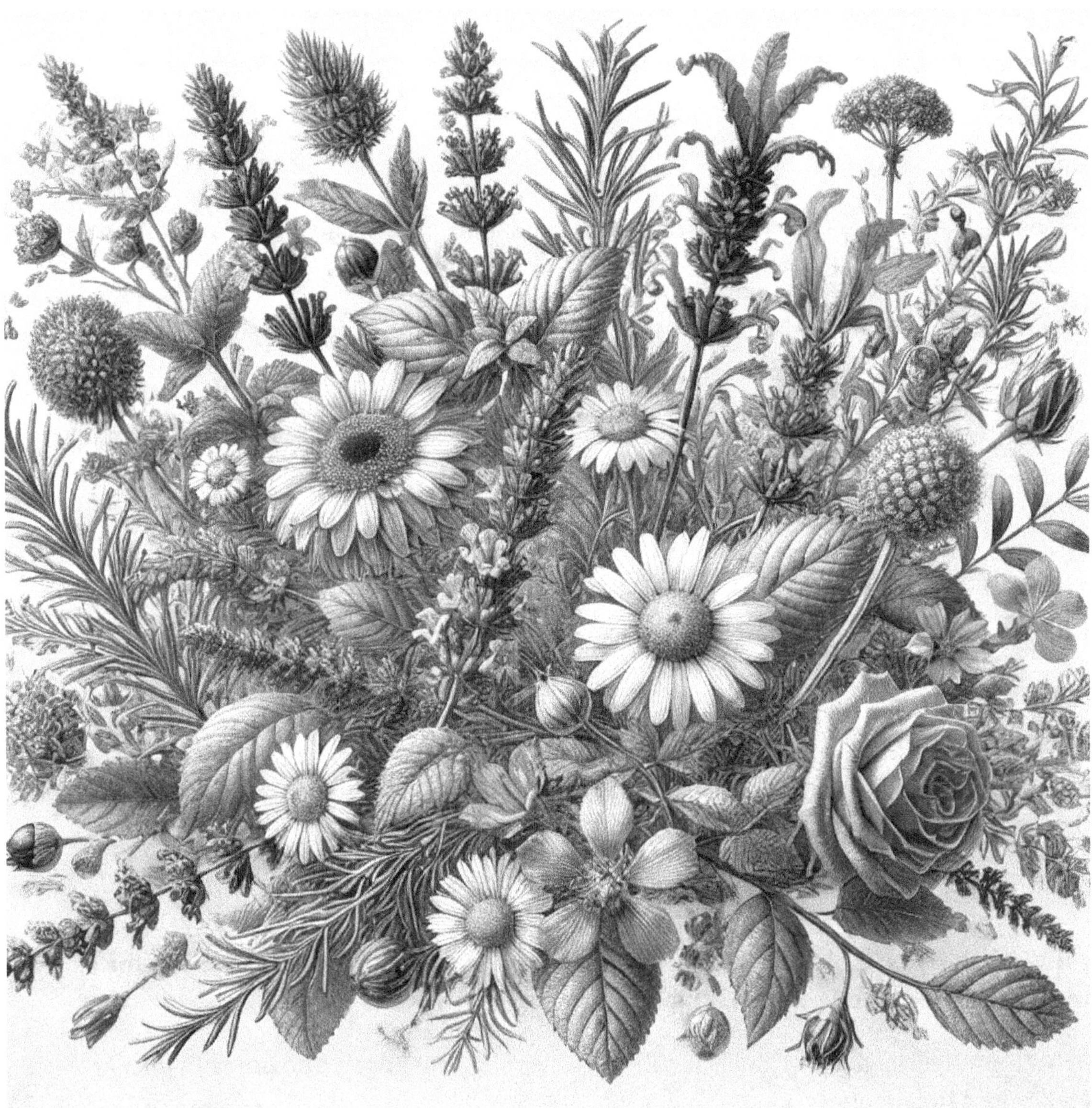

The Power of Nature

For centuries, people have relied on the healing properties of plants and natural ingredients to care for their skin. Let's explore the science behind these powerful botanicals.

A Treasury of Natural Ingredients: Discover a wide range of popular natural ingredients and their benefits:

Hydrators:

Hyaluronic Acid: A powerful humectant that attracts and holds moisture, keeping the skin plump and hydrated.

Aloe Vera: Soothes and calms irritated skin, while also providing hydration and promoting healing.

Glycerine: A humectant that draws moisture from the air and helps to keep the skin hydrated.

Emollients:

Jojoba Oil: Resembles the skin's natural sebum, making it easily absorbed and suitable for all skin types.

Argan Oil: Rich in antioxidants and essential fatty acids, argan oil nourishes and protects the skin.

Sweet Almond Oil: A gentle and nourishing oil that is suitable for even the most sensitive skin.

Antioxidants:

Vitamin C: A powerful antioxidant that protects the skin from environmental damage and promotes collagen production.

Vitamin E: A potent antioxidant that helps to protect the skin from free radical damage and maintain skin elasticity.

Green Tea Extract: Packed with antioxidants, green tea extract helps to protect the skin from environmental stressors and reduce inflammation.

Exfoliants:

AHA (Alpha Hydroxy Acids): Such as lactic acid and glycolic acid, gently exfoliate the skin to remove dead cells and reveal a brighter complexion.

BHA (Beta Hydroxy Acids): Such as salicylic acid, penetrate deep into pores to unclog them and reduce breakouts.

Calming and Soothing:

Chamomile: Soothes irritated skin and reduces inflammation.

Lavender: Calms and relaxes the mind and body while also providing antibacterial and anti-inflammatory benefits.

Calendula: Soothes and heals irritated skin, while also providing antioxidant protection.

Natural vs. Synthetic - A Comparative Analysis:

Natural ingredients: Typically derived from plants, minerals, or other natural sources, often gentler on the skin and less likely to cause irritation.

Synthetic ingredients: Created in a laboratory, may offer certain benefits, but can sometimes be harsh on the skin and may have potential environmental impacts.

The Efficacy of Botanicals: Discover the scientific evidence supporting the efficacy of various botanical ingredients in skincare. Numerous studies have demonstrated the effectiveness of botanical ingredients in addressing a wide range of skin concerns, from hydration and anti-aging to acne and inflammation.

Safety and Allergen Considerations:

Patch Testing: Always perform a patch test on a small area of skin before applying any new ingredient to your face.

Avoid Potential Allergens: Be aware of potential allergens, such as certain essential oils (like citrus oils), and choose ingredients accordingly.

Consult with a Professional: If you have any concerns about potential allergies or sensitivities, consult with a dermatologist or an aromatherapist.

Incorporating New Ingredients - A Step-by-Step Guide:

Start with small amounts: When incorporating a new ingredient, start with a small amount and gradually increase the concentration as needed.

Observe your skin: Monitor your skin's reaction to the new ingredient and adjust the formulation accordingly.

Keep a record: Keep a record of your experiments, noting the ingredients used, the results, and any adjustments made.

Stories of Botanicals

The History of Herbal Remedies: Explore the historical use of botanicals in traditional beauty practices, from ancient Egypt to traditional Chinese medicine. These ancient traditions offer valuable insights into the power of plants and their ability to nourish and heal the skin.

The Science of Botanicals: Discover scientific studies that demonstrate the effectiveness of specific botanical ingredients in addressing various skin concerns. For example, studies have shown that green tea extract can help to protect the skin from UV damage, while tea tree oil has been shown to be effective in reducing acne breakouts.

Key Takeaway

By understanding the science behind natural ingredients, we can harness their power to create effective and nourishing skincare solutions. Exploring the rich history of botanicals and staying informed about the latest scientific research can help us make informed choices and create formulations that truly benefit our skin.

This knowledge empowers us to:

Appreciate the power of nature: Recognize the incredible benefits that nature provides, from the hydrating properties of aloe vera to the antioxidant power of green tea.

Create targeted solutions: Understand how specific ingredients can address specific skin concerns, such as dryness, oiliness, and signs of aging.

Formulate with intention: Combine ingredients synergistically to create formulations that are more effective than any single ingredient alone.

Make informed choices: Select ingredients that are not only effective but also safe, sustainable, and ethically sourced.

By deepening our understanding of the science behind natural ingredients, we can unlock their full potential and create skincare solutions that are both effective and beneficial for our skin and the planet.

The Art of Experimentation

Now that we've explored the science of natural ingredients, let's embrace the spirit of experimentation and discover the joy of creating unique and personalized skincare formulations.

This chapter encourages you to step outside your comfort zone and embrace the creative process. We'll explore how to approach experimentation with curiosity and an open mind, encouraging you to:

Think outside the box - Explore new and innovative ingredient combinations.

Embrace the unknown - Don't be afraid to try new things and see what happens.

Document your process: Keep a record of your experiments, noting the ingredients used, the amounts, and any observations about the texture, scent, and how your skin reacts.

Learn from your mistakes: View any "failures" as learning opportunities and use them to refine your formulations.

By embracing the spirit of experimentation, you'll not only develop your formulation skills but also deepen your understanding of your skin and its unique needs.

Chapter 10: Experimenting with Skincare Formulations

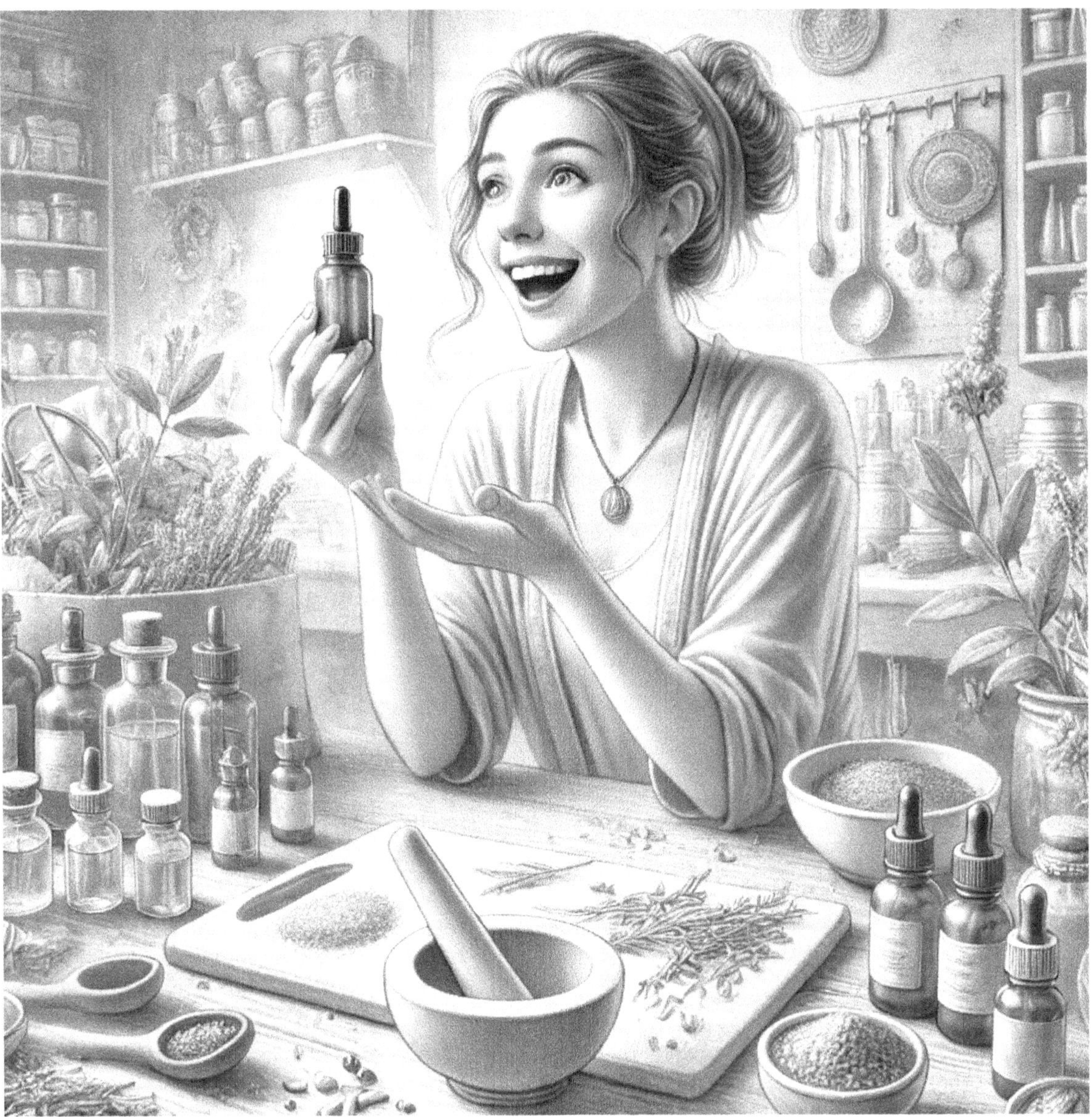

Become Your Own Skincare Scientist

Embrace the spirit of experimentation and discover the joy of creating unique and personalized skincare formulations.

The Importance of Experimentation:

Tailored to Your Needs: Experimentation allows you to fine-tune formulations to perfectly suit your individual skin type and concerns.

Discovering New Favourites: You might stumble upon unexpected ingredient combinations that yield remarkable results.

Building Confidence: Experimentation builds confidence in your ability to create effective and personalized skincare solutions.

Tips for Safe Experimentation:

Start Small: Begin with small batches to avoid wasting ingredients.

Maintain Cleanliness: Ensure all tools and surfaces are clean and sanitized to prevent contamination.

Use High-Quality Ingredients: Choose high-quality, fresh ingredients to ensure the safety and effectiveness of your formulations.

Patch Test: Always perform a patch test on a small area of skin before applying any new formulation to your face.

Documenting Your Journey:

Keep a Skincare Journal: Record your experiments, noting the ingredients used, the amounts, and any observations about the texture, scent, and how your skin reacts.

Take Photos: Take photos of your creations to document your progress and compare results.

Analyse Your Results: Analyse your results and adjust your formulations based on your observations.

Innovations and Trends: Explore emerging trends and innovations in natural skincare:

Superfoods in Skincare: Incorporate nutrient-rich superfoods like berries, seeds, and nuts into your formulations.

Advanced Botanical Extracts: Explore the use of advanced botanical extracts, such as stem cells and plant-derived peptides, for targeted skin concerns.

Probiotics and Prebiotics: Incorporate probiotics and prebiotics to support a healthy skin microbiome.

Encouraging Creativity and Problem-Solving:

Embrace Challenges: View challenges as opportunities to learn and grow. If a formulation doesn't turn out as expected, analyse the results and try again.

Don't Be Afraid to Experiment: Experiment with different textures, scents, and ingredient combinations to discover what works best for you.

Find Inspiration: Find inspiration from nature, other DIY enthusiasts, and the latest research in skincare science.

Stories of Innovation

A Eureka Moment

Sophie, an avid DIY skincare enthusiast, spent countless evenings experimenting with various natural ingredients in her small home laboratory. Her passion for creating effective yet eco-friendly skincare products often led to trial and error, but she was determined to find unique solutions for common skin concerns.

One evening, while working on a moisturizer for dry skin, Sophie decided to combine a hydrating base of aloe vera gel with lightweight oils like rosehip and jojoba. The challenge was finding a natural emulsifier that could seamlessly blend the oil and water-based ingredients. After several failed attempts with beeswax and lecithin, Sophie stumbled upon the idea of incorporating sunflower lecithin—a plant-derived emulsifier often used in cooking. She carefully measured the ingredients and added the lecithin as she heated the mixture.

To her amazement, the formula came together perfectly, creating a lightweight, silky cream that was deeply hydrating yet non-greasy. Excited by her discovery, Sophie tested the product on herself and close friends, who were equally impressed by its performance. Encouraged by their feedback, she refined the formula further, adding a few drops of lavender essential oil for a calming scent.

This "eureka moment" marked a turning point in Sophie's journey. It wasn't just about the successful formulation—it was about the perseverance and creativity that brought it to life. Today, her moisturizing cream is a bestseller in her small skincare line, and she continues to inspire others to embrace experimentation and discover the joy of creating personalized skincare solutions.

Key Takeaway

Experimentation is key to unlocking the full potential of DIY skincare. Embrace the process, learn from your experiences, and enjoy the journey of creating unique and personalized formulations. Remember, every experiment, successful or not, is an opportunity to learn and grow as a DIY skincare enthusiast.

This journey of experimentation is not just about achieving a perfect formula; it's about cultivating a spirit of curiosity and a deeper understanding of your skin. Each experiment, whether successful or not, provides valuable insights into your skin's unique needs and preferences.

Embrace the Learning Process: View each experiment as a learning opportunity. Analyse what worked well and what didn't and adjust your approach accordingly.

Don't Be Afraid to Fail: "Failure" is simply a learning opportunity. Embrace the mistakes, analyse them, and use them to refine your techniques and improve your formulations.

Celebrate Your Successes: Acknowledge and celebrate your successes, no matter how small. Each successful formulation is a testament to your creativity, perseverance, and growing knowledge.

By embracing the process of experimentation and viewing challenges as opportunities for growth, you'll not only develop your formulation skills but also cultivate a deeper connection to your skin and a greater appreciation for the art of creating natural and effective skincare products.

Overcoming Challenges

Even the most seasoned DIY enthusiasts encounter challenges along the way. Whether it's a formulation that separates, an unexpected allergic reaction, or a disappointing result, setbacks are inevitable.

This chapter will explore common challenges encountered in DIY skincare, such as separation, discoloration, and ineffective formulations. We'll delve into the underlying causes of these issues and provide practical troubleshooting strategies to help you overcome them.

By understanding common pitfalls and developing effective troubleshooting techniques, you can navigate the challenges of DIY skincare with confidence and continue to refine your formulations until you achieve the desired results.

This chapter will also emphasize the importance of patience and persistence. Remember that success often comes with practice and perseverance. By embracing the learning process and viewing challenges as opportunities for growth, you can overcome any obstacles and achieve your skincare goals.

Chapter 11: Troubleshooting DIY Skincare Challenges

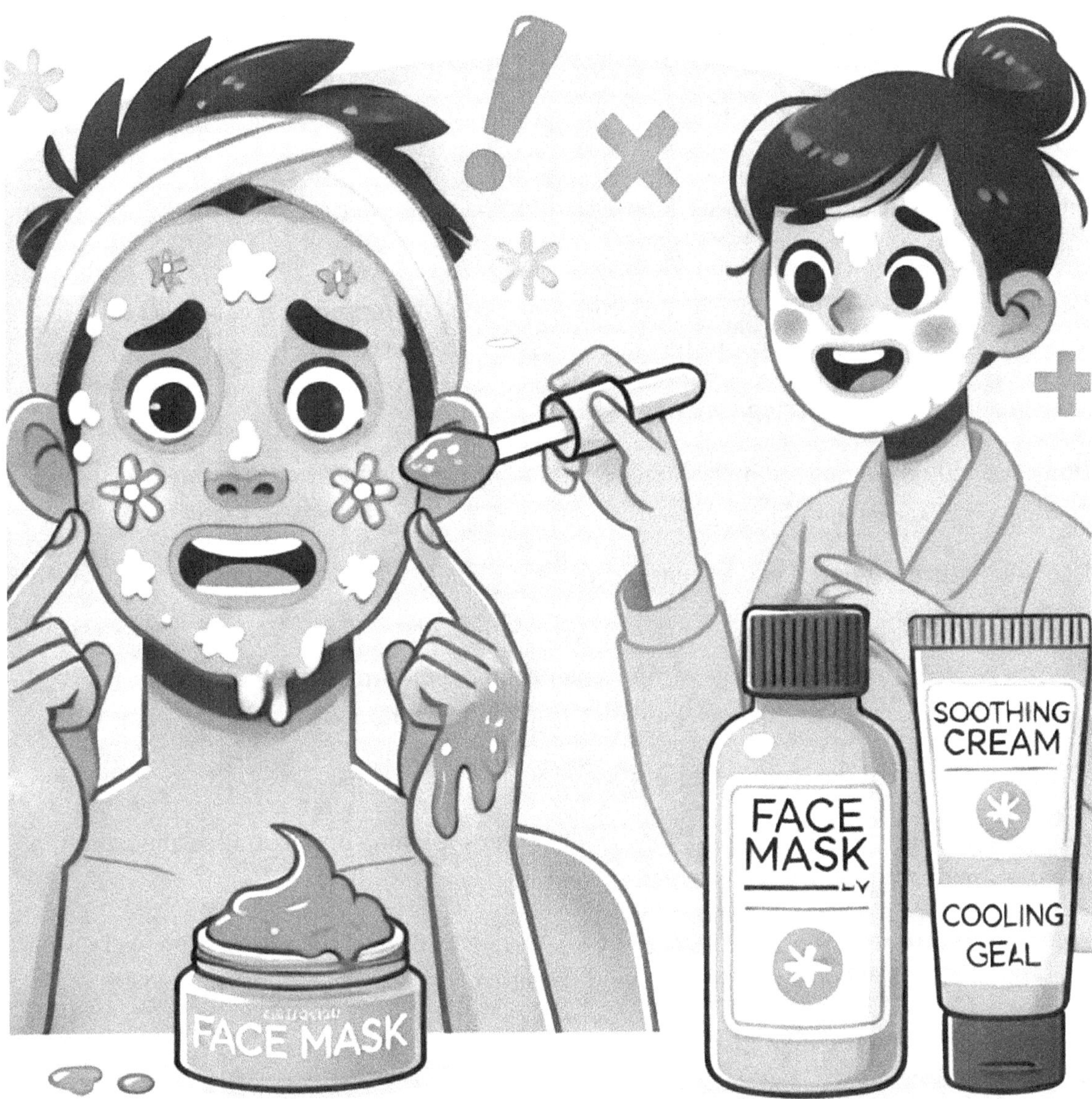

When Things Don't Go According to Plan

Don't worry if your first few attempts don't turn out exactly as expected. Every challenge is an opportunity to learn and grow.

Common Problems and Solutions:

Separation: If your emulsion separates, gently reheat it in a double boiler and stir vigorously until it emulsifies again. You may need to adjust the amount of emulsifier.

Discoloration: Discoloration can occur due to oxidation. Add a few drops of vitamin E oil or a small amount of grapefruit seed extract to help prevent discoloration.

Ineffective Formulations: If your formulation doesn't seem to be providing the desired results, analyse your ingredients and adjust accordingly. Consider adding more potent actives or changing the ratio of ingredients.

Understanding Ingredient Interactions:

Learn about ingredient compatibility: Some ingredients may not be compatible with others and can cause unwanted reactions. Research ingredient interactions before combining them in your formulations.

Consider the order of addition: The order in which you add ingredients can affect the stability and effectiveness of your formulation.

Safe Practices for Resolving Issues:

Don't use mouldy or spoiled ingredients. Discard any ingredients that show signs of spoilage.

If in doubt, throw it out. If you are unsure about the safety of a formulation, discard it rather than risking skin irritation.

Consult reliable resources: If you encounter a problem you can't solve, consult with a knowledgeable formulator or seek guidance from online communities.

The Importance of Patience and Persistence:

Don't get discouraged by setbacks. View challenges as learning opportunities and continue to experiment and refine your formulations.

Embrace the process: Enjoy the journey of experimentation and the satisfaction of creating something beautiful and effective with your own hands.

Building Confidence Through Challenges:

Celebrate your successes: Acknowledge and celebrate your successes, no matter how small.

Learn from your mistakes: Every mistake is an opportunity to learn and improve your skills.

Embrace the learning process: View each challenge as an opportunity to grow and develop your confidence as a DIY skincare enthusiast.

Stories of Triumph

From Mishap to Mastery

"My first attempt at making a DIY face cream was a complete disaster!" recalls Lily, a seasoned DIY enthusiast and advocate for natural skincare. "I meticulously measured out all the ingredients, but when I went to emulsify the oil and water phases, the mixture separated like oil and vinegar. I felt so disheartened! I almost gave up on DIY skincare altogether."

Lily had been inspired by the idea of crafting her own products to avoid synthetic additives and embrace eco-friendly alternatives. Yet, the frustration of failure made her question whether she had the skills to continue. But instead of giving up, Lily decided to treat the setback as a learning opportunity. She consulted online tutorials, read about the science of emulsification, and reached out to a fellow DIYer for advice.

Through her research, Lily discovered a critical mistake: she had used too much water relative to her emulsifier, preventing the ingredients from blending properly. Armed with this new knowledge, she reapproached the task with a more precise plan. This time, she carefully measured her ingredients, adjusted the ratios, and added a small amount of beeswax as a stabilizing emulsifier.

As she stirred the heated mixture, she noticed the ingredients coming together in a smooth, creamy consistency. The satisfaction she felt when the cream emulsified perfectly was overwhelming. "It was such a rewarding feeling to overcome that initial challenge," Lily shares. "It taught me the importance of careful measurement, the value of seeking help when needed, and the power of perseverance."

Since then, Lily has created a range of effective DIY skincare products, from nourishing body balms to soothing lip treatments. Her journey from mishap to mastery has inspired her to share her experiences through workshops and online forums, encouraging others to embrace the learning process. "Now, whenever I encounter a setback, I remember my first failed attempt and approach the challenge with renewed determination," she says. Lily's story is a reminder that every failure is an opportunity to grow, and with patience and persistence, even the most daunting challenges can be overcome.

Key Takeaway

Challenges are an inevitable part of the DIY skincare journey. By developing effective troubleshooting skills and embracing a spirit of perseverance, you can overcome any obstacles and achieve your skincare goals. Remember, every challenge is an opportunity to learn and grow, and the journey of discovery is often more rewarding than the destination.

This journey is not always a linear path. You will encounter setbacks, experience frustrations, and perhaps even experience some less-than-stellar results. However, these challenges are valuable learning experiences. They help you understand your skin better, refine your formulation techniques, and develop the resilience and problem-solving skills necessary to succeed in your DIY skincare endeavours.

By embracing the learning process and viewing challenges as opportunities for growth, you can cultivate a sense of resilience and develop the confidence to overcome any obstacles that may arise. Remember, every successful DIYer has faced challenges along the way.

Embrace the journey, learn from your experiences, and celebrate your successes, no matter how small.

The Power of Community

The journey of eco-friendly skincare is more enriching when shared with others. Connecting with a community of like-minded individuals can provide valuable support, inspiration, and a wealth of shared knowledge.

This chapter will explore the power of community in fostering a sense of belonging, sharing knowledge, and driving collective action. We'll discuss the importance of connecting with other DIY enthusiasts, both online and offline, and how these connections can enrich your skincare journey.

By sharing your experiences, learning from others, and collaborating with fellow DIYers, you can create a supportive network that fosters creativity, encourages growth, and drives collective action towards a more sustainable and fulfilling future.

Chapter 12: Building a Community Around Eco-Friendly Skincare

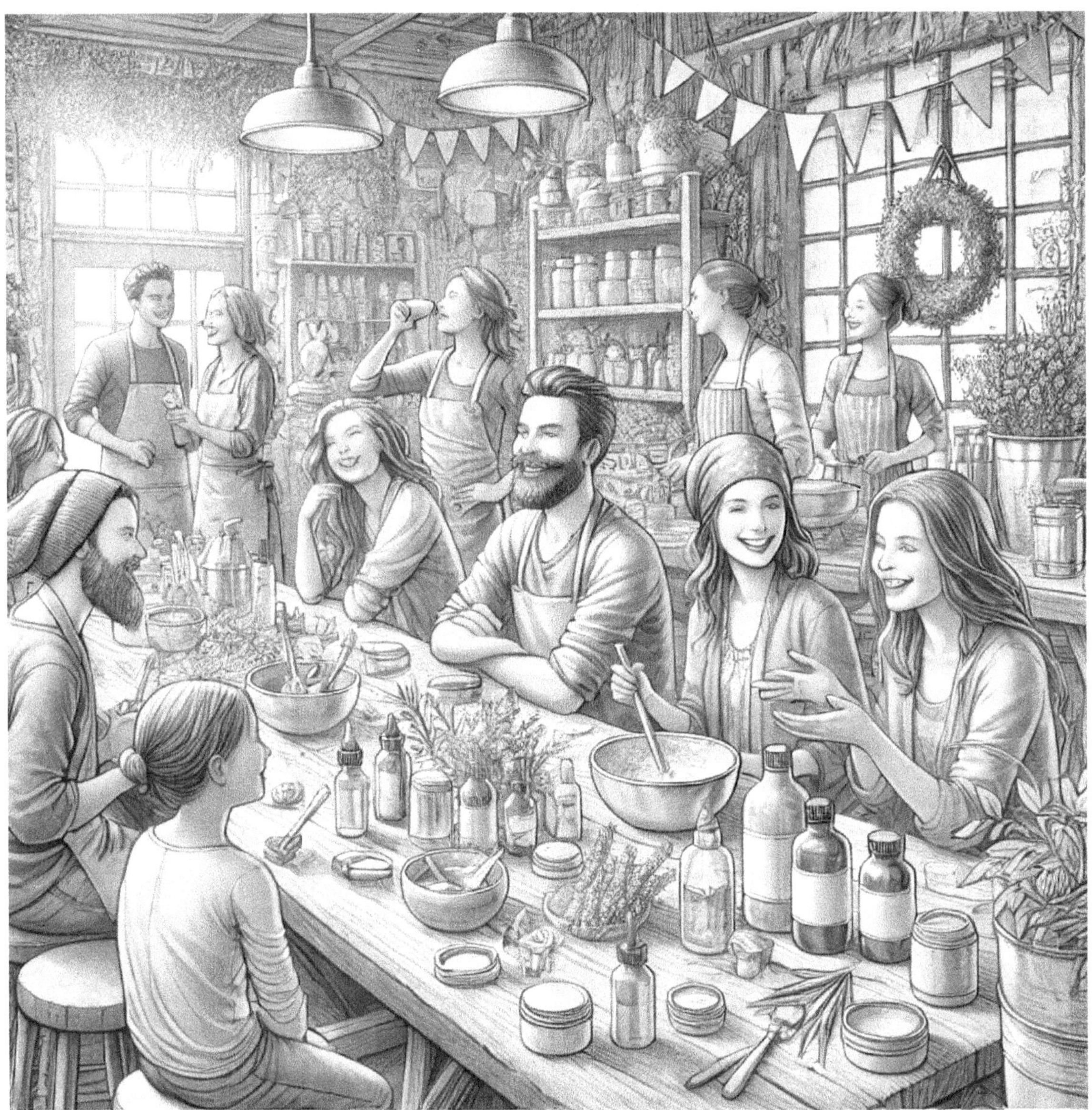

The Power of Connection

Connecting with others who share your passion for eco-friendly skincare can provide valuable support, inspiration, and a wealth of shared knowledge.

The Importance of Community:

Shared Experiences: Connecting with others who share your passion for eco-friendly skincare can provide a sense of belonging and shared understanding.

Support and Encouragement: Sharing your experiences and challenges with others can provide valuable support and encouragement, reminding you that you are not alone on your journey.

Access to Knowledge and Resources: Connecting with other DIY enthusiasts can provide access to a wealth of knowledge and resources, from ingredient recommendations and formulation tips to information about sustainable living.

Inspiration and Motivation: Seeing the successes and inspiring journeys of others can motivate you to continue your own path and strive for greater things.

Finding Your Tribe - Local and Online Communities:

Local Workshops and Events: Attend workshops, classes, and meetups focused on DIY skincare, herbalism, and sustainable living. These events provide opportunities to connect with other enthusiasts in your local area.

Online Forums and Groups: Join online forums and social media groups dedicated to eco-friendly skincare, DIY beauty, and sustainable living. These platforms provide a space for sharing information, asking questions, and connecting with people from around the world.

Social media: Utilize social media platforms like Instagram and Pinterest to connect with other DIY enthusiasts, share your creations, and follow inspiring accounts.

Sharing Experiences and Tips:

Share your knowledge: Share your knowledge and experiences with others through blog posts, social media, or by teaching workshops.

Learn from others: Actively listen to the experiences and insights of other DIY enthusiasts and learn from their successes and challenges.

Provide constructive feedback: Offer constructive feedback and support to other members of the community.

Collaborative Opportunities:

Organize local events: Collaborate with other DIY enthusiasts to organize local events, such as workshops, swaps, and potlucks.

Support local businesses: Support local businesses that prioritize sustainability and ethical practices.

Advocate for change: Advocate for policies and initiatives that support sustainable living and environmental protection.

Building a Supportive Network:

Connect with like-minded individuals: Cultivate relationships with other DIY enthusiasts who inspire and motivate you.

Create a supportive environment: Foster a sense of community and support among your fellow DIYers, celebrating each other's successes and offering encouragement during challenges.

Stories of Community

A Community-Driven Initiative

In the heart of a bustling city, a group of passionate DIY skincare enthusiasts decided to transform their shared love for natural beauty into a larger movement. They organized "Bloom," a vibrant, day-long celebration dedicated to sustainable living and eco-conscious beauty practices. Their goal was simple: to bring people together, raise awareness about sustainable choices, and inspire others to embrace a more environmentally friendly lifestyle.

Bloom offered a variety of engaging activities; each designed to educate and empower attendees. Workshops included hands-on natural skincare formulation classes, herbalism demonstrations that highlighted the healing power of plants, and zero-waste living seminars offering practical tips for reducing household waste. Local vendors showcased their eco-friendly goods, from handcrafted soaps and natural balms to sustainable clothing and upcycled home decor.

The event also featured community-focused activities to ensure everyone felt welcome. A designated area for children offered fun, educational activities like planting seeds and crafting with recyclable materials. Meanwhile, live music and food trucks serving delicious plant-based cuisine created a lively and inclusive atmosphere.

Bloom turned out to be a resounding success, drawing hundreds of attendees from diverse backgrounds. The event not only highlighted sustainable beauty practices but also fostered a deep sense of connection among participants. Many left with not only new knowledge but also a commitment to adopting eco-conscious habits in their own lives. By the end of the day, Bloom had sparked a ripple effect, inspiring local businesses to adopt greener practices and community members to continue championing sustainability.

The Power of Shared Knowledge

Sarah, a curious but overwhelmed newcomer to DIY skincare, initially struggled to navigate the vast amount of information available online. Conflicting advice about ingredients, formulations, and techniques left her feeling paralyzed and unsure of where to begin. Discouraged but not ready to give up, Sarah decided to join an online community dedicated to eco-friendly skincare.

To her delight, she found a welcoming space filled with experienced DIYers eager to share their knowledge. Members of the community answered her questions with patience and encouragement, offering insights on everything from choosing high-quality ingredients to troubleshooting common issues like product separation. Sarah also learned the importance of patch testing and tailoring formulations to her individual skin needs.

With the community's support, Sarah's confidence blossomed. She began experimenting with her own formulations, starting with a simple lavender-infused face oil. Encouraged by her success, she progressed to crafting more complex products, like serums and balms. Along the way, she discovered a profound joy in the creative process and a deeper appreciation for the science behind natural skincare.

Today, Sarah is an active member of the same community that guided her journey. She shares her experiences and offers advice to newcomers, paying forward the support she once received. Her story illustrates the incredible power of community to foster learning, build confidence, and ignite passions.

Key Takeaways

These stories showcase the transformative impact of collective action and shared knowledge. Whether through large-scale events like Bloom or smaller online communities, the power of connection cannot be overstated. By coming together, individuals and groups can:

Foster a Sense of Belonging: Events like Bloom and online forums provide spaces where people can feel supported and inspired.

Share Knowledge and Expertise: Communities help newcomers navigate challenges, offering guidance that might otherwise take years to learn.

Drive Collective Action: When individuals unite around a common goal, their combined efforts can create meaningful, lasting change.

Through community-driven initiatives and the exchange of knowledge, we can build a more sustainable, inclusive, and empowering future—one where individual actions contribute to a larger movement for positive change.

Chapter 13: Lifelong Learning in Eco-Friendly Skincare

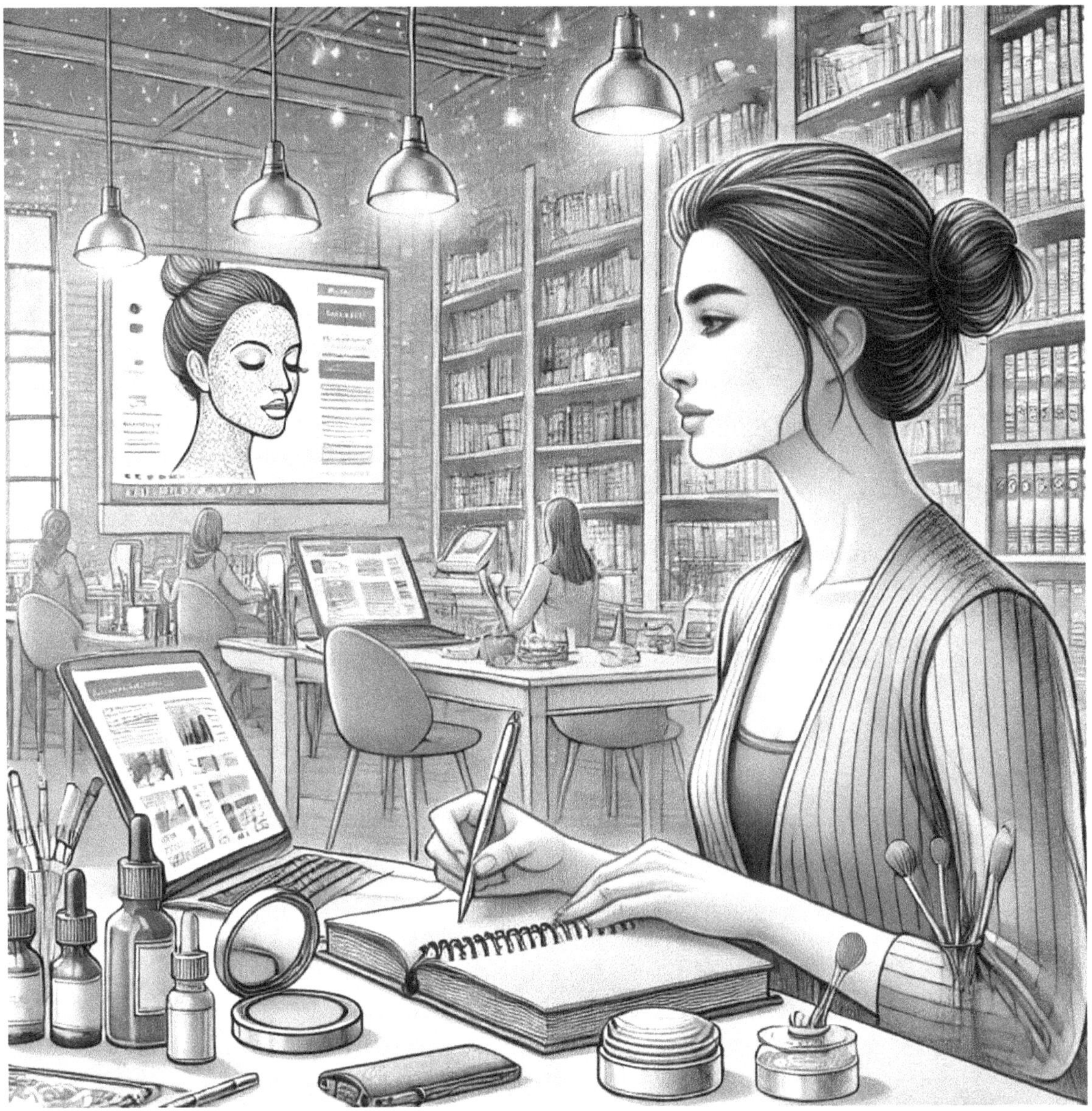

The Never-Ending Journey of Discovery

Embrace the spirit of lifelong learning and continue to expand your knowledge and skills in the ever-evolving world of eco-friendly skincare.

Staying Informed:

Follow industry leaders: Follow blogs, websites, and social media accounts of experts in the field of natural skincare and sustainability.

Read books and articles: Stay updated on the latest research, trends, and innovations in skincare science and sustainability.

Subscribe to newsletters: Subscribe to newsletters from your favourite brands, industry publications, and environmental organizations.

Enriching Your Knowledge: Workshops and Courses:

Attend workshops and classes: Participate in workshops and classes on topics such as botanical skincare, aromatherapy, and sustainable business practices.

Online courses: Explore online courses and certifications in areas such as herbalism, aromatherapy, and natural skincare formulation.

Seek mentorship: Connect with experienced mentors in the field of natural skincare and sustainable living.

Cultivating Curiosity and Exploration:

Ask questions: Never stop asking questions and seeking new information.

Embrace experimentation: Continuously experiment with new ingredients, formulations, and techniques.

Challenge your assumptions: Be open to new ideas and willing to challenge your existing beliefs.

Adapting to Change:

Stay informed about evolving trends: Keep up to date on the latest trends and innovations in the field of eco-friendly skincare.

Adapt your practices: Be willing to adapt your practices and knowledge as the field of eco-friendly skincare continues to evolve.

Embrace sustainability as a journey: Recognize that sustainability is an ongoing journey and strive for continuous improvement in all areas of your life.

Stories of Continuous Learning

A Journey of Self-Improvement

Amelia, a dedicated DIY enthusiast, embodies the spirit of lifelong learning. Her passion for creating natural skincare products began as a simple hobby but has since evolved into an ever-deepening journey of self-discovery and improvement. With an insatiable curiosity, Amelia continually seeks to expand her knowledge and refine her craft.

She regularly attends local workshops on herbalism and aromatherapy, where she learns about the therapeutic properties of plants and essential oils. These hands-on sessions not only teach her new techniques but also allow her to connect with like-minded individuals who share her commitment to sustainable living. Beyond in-person workshops, Amelia dives into online courses on natural skincare formulation, mastering advanced concepts like emulsification, ingredient stability, and pH balancing.

Amelia's thirst for knowledge extends to scientific research. She avidly reads articles and studies on botanical ingredients, keeping herself informed about the latest breakthroughs in skincare science. This habit has helped her understand the mechanisms behind her formulations, from the antioxidant properties of green tea to the hydrating power of hyaluronic acid.

Her meticulous approach is central to her success. Amelia maintains a detailed journal where she documents every experiment—recording ingredient ratios, methods, and her observations on texture, scent, and effectiveness. By analyzing these results, she identifies areas for improvement and adapts her recipes to suit her changing skin needs. When an experiment fails, she views it as an opportunity to learn, tweaking her process until she achieves the desired outcome.

"I've learned so much through continuous learning," Amelia shares. "Every workshop, every article, every failed experiment has taught me something new. This journey of self-improvement has not only improved my skincare routine but also fostered a deeper appreciation for the power of nature and the importance of lifelong learning."

Amelia's dedication to growth and innovation has transformed her DIY skincare practice into an art form. Her journey serves as an inspiration, reminding us that the pursuit of knowledge is not just about achieving perfection but about embracing the process of learning, evolving, and connecting with the world around us. Through her tireless efforts, Amelia has discovered that the path to self-improvement is as rewarding as the results it produces.

Key Takeaway

Embrace the journey of continuous learning, and never stop exploring the fascinating world of eco-friendly skincare. By staying informed, expanding your knowledge, and adapting to change, you can continue to grow and evolve as an eco-conscious individual and contribute to a more sustainable future.

This journey of self-discovery extends beyond personal benefit. By sharing your knowledge and experiences with others, you can inspire and motivate them to embrace sustainable practices and contribute to a broader movement towards a more sustainable and equitable future.

Sharing Your Eco-Friendly Journey

Sharing your passion for eco-friendly skincare with others can inspire and motivate them to embrace sustainable practices. Let's explore the power of sharing your journey and how you can contribute to a larger movement towards a more sustainable and beautiful world.

This chapter will delve into the importance of sharing your experiences, knowledge, and creations with others. We'll explore various platforms for sharing your journey, from blogging and social media to workshops and community events.

Furthermore, we'll discuss the power of storytelling and how to craft compelling narratives that resonate with your audience and inspire them to embrace eco-friendly living. By sharing your passion and inspiring others, you can contribute to a broader movement towards sustainable beauty and create a positive impact on the world.

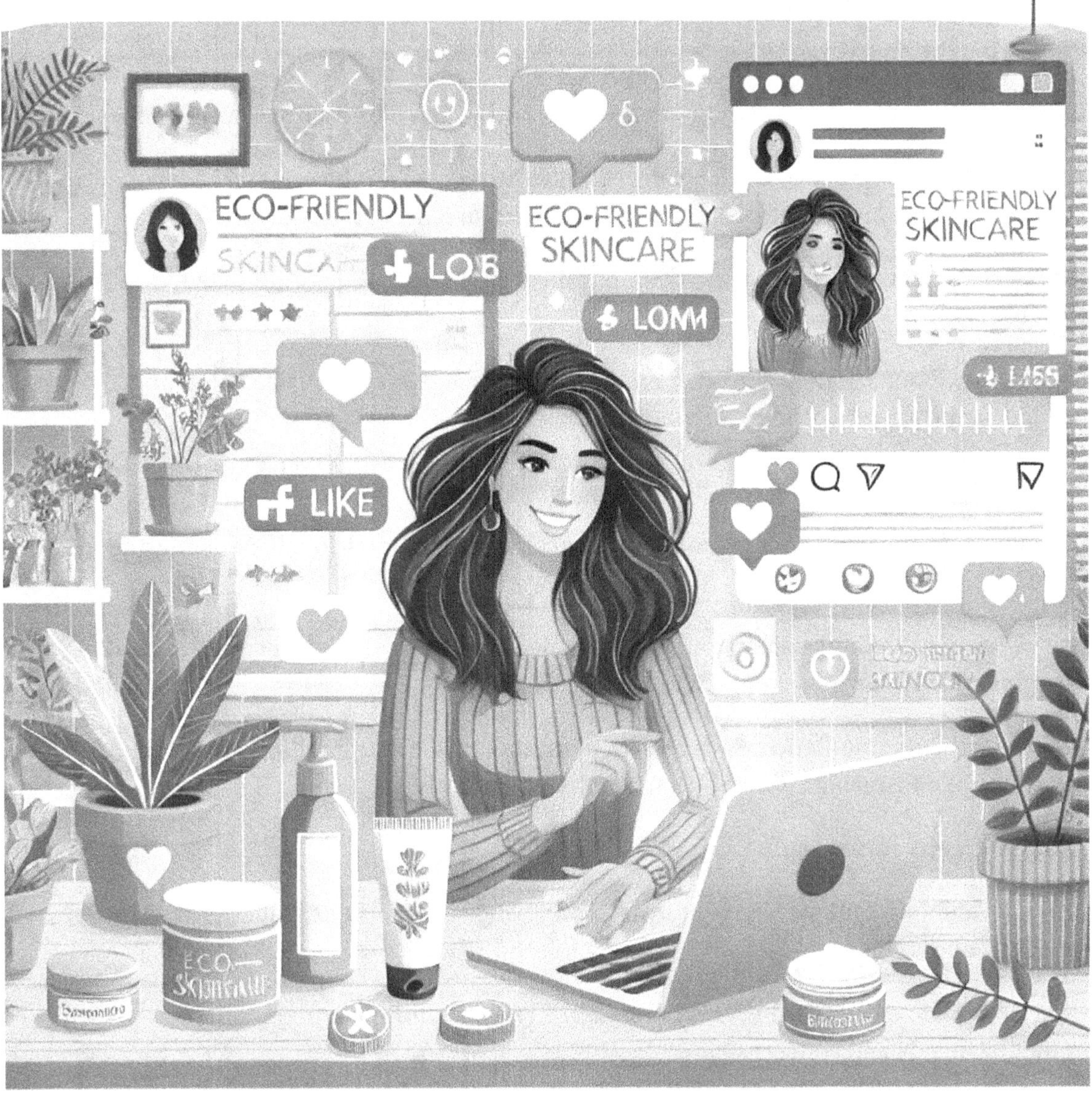

Inspiring Others Through Sharing

Sharing your experiences, knowledge, and creations can inspire others to embrace eco-friendly skincare and contribute to a more sustainable future.

The Importance of Sharing:

Inspiring Others: Share your successes and challenges to inspire others to embark on their own eco-friendly skincare journeys.

Raising Awareness: Raise awareness about the importance of sustainable living and the impact of individual choices on the environment.

Creating a Ripple Effect: Your actions can inspire others to make conscious choices and contribute to a broader movement towards sustainability.

Platforms for Sharing:

Blogging: Share your knowledge and experiences through a blog or online journal.

Social media: Utilize social media platforms like Instagram, Pinterest, and Facebook to share your creations, connect with other enthusiasts, and inspire your followers.

Workshops and Classes: Teach workshops and classes to share your knowledge and skills with others.

Community Events: Participate in community events and share your passion for eco-friendly skincare with others.

The Power of Storytelling:

Craft compelling stories: Share your experiences and insights through engaging and relatable stories.

Use visuals: Utilize high-quality photos and videos to capture the beauty and appeal of your creations.

Connect with your audience: Engage with your audience by responding to comments and questions and fostering a sense of community.

Engaging Your Audience:

Provide valuable content: Share informative and engaging content that educates and inspires your audience.

Offer personalized advice: Provide personalized advice and recommendations based on individual needs and concerns.

Create a sense of community: Foster a sense of community among your followers by encouraging them to share their experiences and connect with each other.

Stories of Inspiration

A Blogger's Impact:

Meet Elena, a passionate DIYer who turned her love for natural skincare into a thriving online community. She started a blog to document her skincare journey, sharing her recipes, tips, and experiences with her readers.

Initially, Elena's blog was a personal outlet, a way to share her passion with friends and family. However, as she consistently shared high-quality content, her audience began to grow. She connected with other DIY enthusiasts, answered their questions, and provided personalized advice.

Elena's blog became a valuable resource for those seeking to embrace eco-friendly skincare. She inspired her followers to experiment with natural ingredients, embrace sustainable practices, and connect with their own creativity. Her influence extended beyond her blog, inspiring many to embark on their own DIY skincare journeys and contribute to a more sustainable beauty movement.

Community-Driven Change:

In a small coastal town, a group of concerned citizens noticed a growing problem with plastic pollution on their local beaches. Recognizing the impact of plastic packaging on the environment, they decided to act.

Inspired by the growing movement towards zero-waste living, they organized a community event called "Plastic-Free Beauty," inviting local businesses, DIY enthusiasts, and community members to participate. The event featured workshops on creating natural skincare products, demonstrations on reducing plastic waste in the bathroom, and a swap meet where participants could exchange unwanted beauty products.

The event was a resounding success, bringing together the community and raising awareness about the environmental impact of the beauty industry. Inspired by the event's success, the community continued to organize similar initiatives, advocating for local businesses to adopt more sustainable practices and inspiring residents to make conscious choices in their daily lives.

These stories highlight the power of sharing experiences, inspiring others, and fostering a sense of community. By connecting with others and sharing our knowledge, we can create a powerful movement that drives positive change and contributes to a more sustainable and equitable future for all.

Key Takeaway

By sharing your journey and inspiring others, you can contribute to a broader movement towards sustainable beauty and create a positive impact on the world. Remember, every action, no matter how small, can make a difference.

Your individual choices, from the products you choose to the way you share your knowledge, have the power to influence others and contribute to a larger movement towards sustainability. By embracing eco-conscious practices in your own life and inspiring others to do the same, you become part of a collective effort to create a more sustainable and equitable future for all.

Eco-Friendly Skincare: A Path to Global Sustainability

Our individual skincare choices have a ripple effect that extends far beyond our personal routines. Every product we choose, every ingredient we support, and every package we discard contributes to the collective impact on our planet. This chapter explores the intersection of eco-friendly skincare practices and global sustainability efforts, highlighting the powerful role individuals and industries play in shaping a more sustainable future.

The Beauty Industry's Environmental Impact

The beauty industry, though dedicated to enhancing personal well-being, has significant environmental consequences. Key challenges include:

Plastic Pollution: With billions of plastic containers produced annually, much of the beauty industry's packaging ends up in landfills or the ocean. Single-use plastics, often non-recyclable, contribute to the growing problem of microplastic pollution that threatens marine life and ecosystems.

Water Scarcity: Many conventional beauty products require vast amounts of water during production. Additionally, water-based formulations increase industry's reliance on this finite resource, exacerbating global water scarcity.

Deforestation: The extraction of natural ingredients like palm oil and certain essential oils often leads to deforestation, loss of biodiversity, and habitat destruction for endangered species.

These challenges demand urgent action from both businesses and consumers to mitigate their impact on the environment.

The Power of Conscious Consumerism

As consumers, our choices hold tremendous power. By prioritizing eco-friendly practices in our skincare routines, we can help drive meaningful change. Here are a few ways individuals can make a difference:

Choose Sustainable Products: Look for brands that use biodegradable, recyclable, or refillable packaging. Opt for products that are waterless or use minimal water in their formulations.

Support Ethical Brands: Research companies that prioritize sustainability and transparency. Brands that use ethically sourced ingredients and actively work to reduce their carbon footprint deserve our support.

Embrace Zero-Waste Practices: Transition to reusable cotton pads, compostable tools, and bulk purchasing to minimize waste. Small, conscious changes add up to a significant collective impact.

Educate and Advocate: Share knowledge about sustainable practices with others and encourage them to make informed choices. Awareness is the first step toward action.

The Role of Collective Action

While individual actions are vital, the scale of environmental challenges necessitates collaboration on a larger scale. Businesses, consumers, and environmental organizations must come together to create lasting change.

Cross-Industry Collaboration: The formation of alliances, like the Sustainable Beauty Alliance, has proven that competitors can unite to address shared challenges. By establishing industry-wide standards for sustainability, businesses can collectively reduce their environmental footprint.

Environmental Advocacy: Organizations like Greenpeace and the World Wildlife Fund (WWF) partner with beauty brands to promote responsible ingredient sourcing, reduce deforestation, and lobby for policy changes that support sustainability.

Innovation and Investment: Companies are investing in groundbreaking solutions, such as biodegradable packaging, lab-grown ingredients to replace environmentally harmful ones, and carbon-neutral supply chains. These innovations represent the future of a sustainable beauty industry.

A Vision for the Future

The interconnectedness of our actions and their global impact cannot be overstated. By embracing eco-friendly skincare practices, we align our personal choices with broader sustainability goals. Together, as individuals and as a global community, we can address pressing environmental challenges and create a beauty industry that is not only beautiful but also responsible and equitable.

This chapter is a call to action for consumers, businesses, and environmental organizations alike. By working together, we can transform the beauty industry into a force for good—one that supports the well-being of people and the planet for generations to come. Through conscious consumerism, collective action, and a commitment to innovation, we can contribute to a future where sustainability is the foundation of beauty.

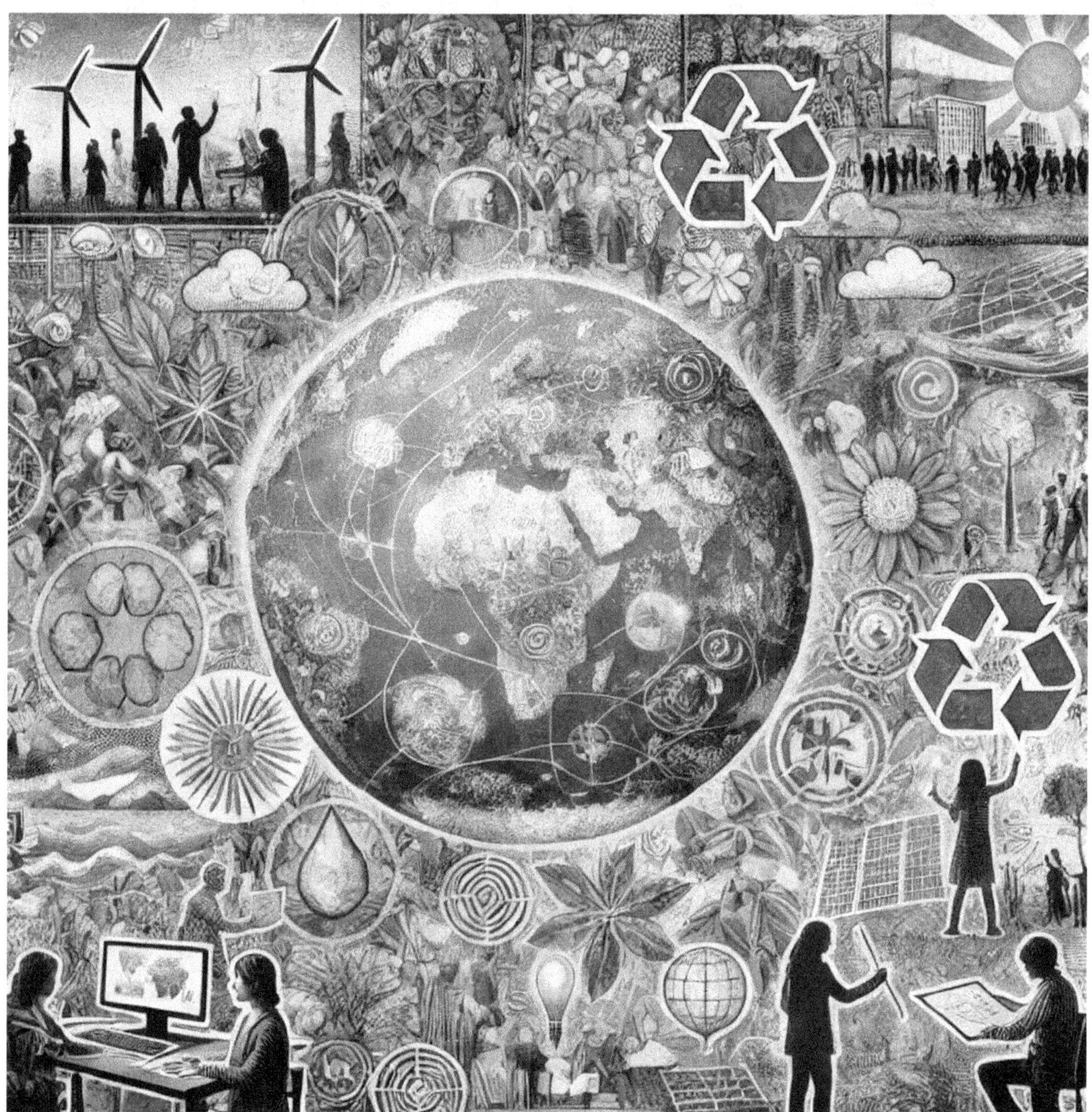

A Global Perspective

Eco-friendly skincare is not just about personal well-being; it's about contributing to a larger movement towards global sustainability.

Understanding Global Sustainability:

The Three Pillars of Sustainability: Explore the three pillars of sustainability: environmental protection, social equity, and economic viability.

Interconnectedness: Understand how environmental, social, and economic factors are interconnected and interdependent.

Global Challenges: Recognize the global challenges facing humanity, such as climate change, poverty, and inequality.

The Role of Conscious Consumerism:

Making Informed Choices: Understand the power of conscious consumerism and how your purchasing decisions can impact the environment, society, and the economy.

Supporting Sustainable Brands: Choose to support brands that prioritize sustainability, ethical sourcing, and fair labour practices.

Reducing Your Ecological Footprint: Minimize your environmental impact by reducing waste, conserving resources, and embracing sustainable living practices.

Connecting the Dots - Individual Choices and Global Impact:

The Ripple Effect: Explore how your individual skincare choices, from sourcing ingredients to minimizing waste, can have a ripple effect, influencing the behaviour of others and contributing to broader sustainability efforts.

Collective Action: Recognize that collective action is essential to address global sustainability challenges. By working together, we can create a more sustainable and equitable future for all.

Cross-Industry Collaboration:

Partnerships for Change: Explore the importance of cross-industry collaboration in driving sustainability efforts, such as partnerships between businesses, NGOs, and government agencies.

Innovation and Collaboration: Encourage innovation and collaboration within the beauty industry to develop more sustainable and eco-friendly products and practices.

The Future of Sustainable Beauty - A Vision for the Future:

A Circular Economy: Envision a future where the beauty industry operates within a circular economy, with minimal waste and maximum resource utilization.

Regenerative Practices: Support brands that prioritize regenerative practices, such as supporting local communities, restoring ecosystems, and minimizing their environmental impact.

Empowering Individuals: Empower individuals to make informed choices and become active participants in the transition to a more sustainable future.

Stories of Global Impact

A Global Initiative - Making a Difference on a Worldwide Scale:

Imagine a global network of beauty brands, NGOs, and environmental organizations united by a shared vision: a sustainable and equitable beauty industry. This is the driving force behind "Global Beauty for Good," a groundbreaking initiative that empowers communities around the world.

Global Beauty for Good focuses on:

Supporting local artisans and cooperatives: Providing fair wages and sustainable livelihoods to communities in developing countries by sourcing ingredients ethically and supporting local businesses.

Investing in regenerative agriculture: Supporting sustainable farming practices that restore biodiversity, protect ecosystems, and improve soil health.

Empowering women and girls: Providing educational opportunities and vocational training to women and girls in underprivileged communities, empowering them to become leaders in the beauty industry.

Reducing environmental impact: Implementing industry-wide standards for sustainable packaging, minimizing waste, and reducing carbon emissions throughout the supply chain.

Global Beauty for Good serves as a powerful example of how collective action can create meaningful change on a global scale. By uniting diverse stakeholders and leveraging their collective strengths, this initiative is driving positive impact across the globe.

A Community-Driven Movement - Inspiring Change from the Ground Up:

In a small village in Southeast Asia, a group of women artisans, struggling to find sustainable livelihoods, discovered the power of natural beauty. With the support of a local NGO, they began to cultivate and harvest local botanicals, creating handcrafted skincare products using traditional techniques.

Word of their unique and effective products spread, attracting the attention of a fair-trade organization. Through this partnership, the women's cooperative gained access to new markets, fair wages, and opportunities for skill development.

This community-driven initiative not only empowered local women but also showcased the potential of sustainable and ethical beauty practices. It inspired other communities to explore similar initiatives, demonstrating the power of grassroots efforts in driving positive change within the beauty industry.

These stories highlight the importance of collective action and the power of individual voices in creating a more sustainable and equitable future. By working together and embracing a spirit of collaboration, we can create a beauty industry that is both beautiful and beneficial for the planet and its people.

Key Takeaway

By sharing your journey and inspiring others, you can contribute to a broader movement towards sustainable beauty and create a positive impact on the world. Remember, every action, no matter how small, can make a difference.

Your individual choices, from the products you choose to the way you share your knowledge, have the power to influence others and contribute to a larger movement towards sustainability. By embracing eco-conscious practices in your own life and inspiring others to do the same, you become part of a collective effort to create a more sustainable and equitable future for all.

This is more than just about personal well-being; it's about recognizing our interconnectedness with the planet and taking responsibility for our impact.

A Global Perspective

Our individual skincare choices have a profound impact on the planet. Let's explore how eco-friendly skincare practices intersect with global sustainability efforts.

This chapter will delve into the interconnectedness of our individual actions and the global challenges facing our planet. We'll examine how the beauty industry contributes to environmental issues, such as plastic pollution, water scarcity, and deforestation.

Furthermore, we'll discuss the power of conscious consumerism and how our individual choices can make a significant difference. By choosing sustainable products, supporting ethical brands, and embracing zero-waste practices, we can contribute to a more sustainable and equitable future for all.

This chapter will also explore the importance of collective action and the role of cross-industry collaboration in driving positive change within the beauty industry. By working together, businesses, consumers, and environmental organizations can create a more sustainable and beautiful future for generations to come.

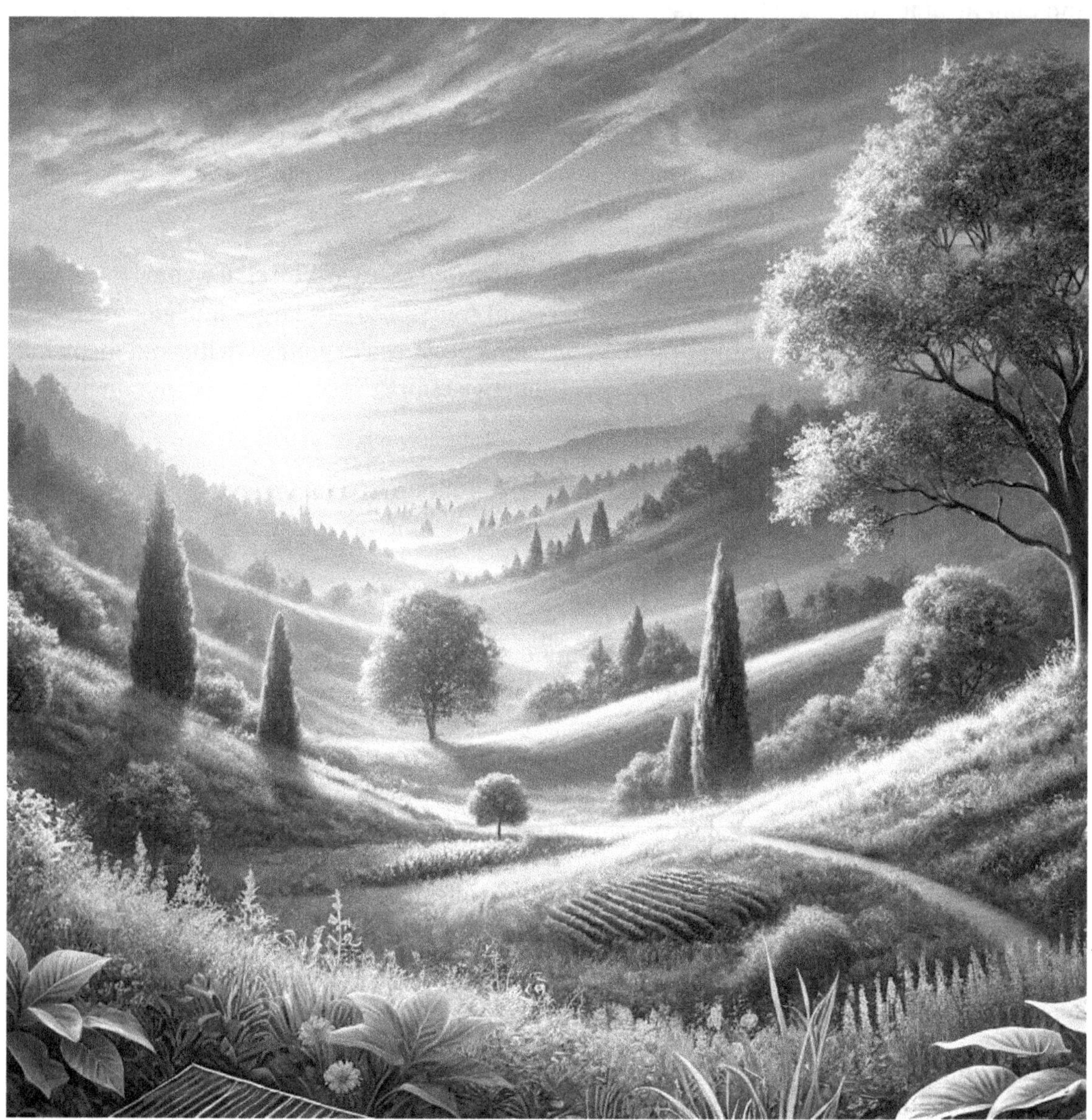

A New Beginning

This book has been a journey of exploration, discovery, and empowerment. We've delved into the science of skin biology, mastered the art of formulating natural skincare products, explored the importance of sustainability, and discovered the power of community.

A Reflection and a Path Forward

Recap of Key Lessons - Reflect on the key lessons learned throughout this journey:

The importance of understanding your skin's unique needs.

The power of natural ingredients.

The benefits of DIY skincare.

The importance of sustainability in all aspects of life.

The power of community and collective action.

Setting Sustainability Goals: Set personal and community sustainability goals.

Reduce your environmental impact: Minimize your waste, conserve resources, and choose sustainable transportation options.

Support local businesses: Support local businesses that prioritize sustainability and ethical practices.

Get involved in your community: Participate in community events and advocate for environmental protection.

Celebrating Successes and Milestones: Celebrate your achievements, both big and small, and acknowledge the progress you've made on your eco-friendly skincare journey.

A Vision for the Future: Envision a future where sustainability is the cornerstone of the beauty industry, where individuals embrace conscious choices, and where we all work together to create a healthier planet for future generations.

A Call to Action: This is not just a goodbye; it's a farewell until our next adventure in the world of sustainable beauty. Continue to explore, learn, and grow as you embrace a life of eco-conscious living.

Stories of Inspiration

A Personal Reflection:

My own journey into eco-friendly skincare has been a winding path filled with both triumphs and challenges. It began with a simple desire for healthier skin, but quickly evolved into a deeper exploration of sustainability and my own impact on the planet.

I remember my initial attempts at DIY skincare – messy experiments in my kitchen, countless failed formulations, and the occasional skin irritation. Yet, each setback was an opportunity to learn. I meticulously documented my experiments, analysing what worked and what didn't. I consulted online resources, joined online communities, and even attended a local workshop on herbalism.

Over time, my formulations improved, my understanding of skin biology deepened, and my passion for sustainable living grew. This journey has not only transformed my skincare routine but also inspired me to make more conscious choices in all aspects of my life. It has taught me the importance of perseverance, the power of community, and the profound impact that individual actions can have on the world.

A Busy Professional's Transformative Journey

Emily, a busy professional juggling the demands of work and life, initially approached the idea of eco-friendly skincare with skepticism. Overwhelmed by the sheer volume of information available and unsure where to start, she felt that adopting sustainable practices might be too complicated or time-consuming for her lifestyle.

Her perspective began to shift after she stumbled upon this book and connected with a supportive online community of eco-conscious individuals. Encouraged by their advice and success stories, Emily decided to take the first step on her journey toward sustainability.

She started small, incorporating a few manageable changes into her routine. She replaced her conventional cleanser with a natural, eco-friendly alternative and switched to reusable cotton rounds instead of disposable ones. These simple swaps proved to be effective and easy to maintain, giving her the confidence to explore further.

As Emily became more comfortable, she began experimenting with DIY skincare formulations. She crafted a gentle, homemade exfoliating scrub using oatmeal and honey and discovered the joys of working with sustainable ingredients like shea butter and essential oils. Each success fueled her enthusiasm and deepened her commitment to eco-friendly practices.

Her skincare transformation soon sparked a broader shift in her lifestyle. Emily became more mindful of her overall consumption habits, actively reducing her reliance on single-use plastics and choosing products with minimal or compostable packaging. She started supporting local businesses, purchasing ingredients from nearby farmers' markets, and participating in community initiatives focused on environmental protection.

Emily's journey didn't stop there. Inspired by her progress, she began advocating for sustainability within her workplace, encouraging colleagues to adopt small but impactful changes, like recycling and reducing energy usage. Her story is a testament to the ripple effect that individual actions can have on the broader community.

"By embracing eco-friendly skincare practices, I've not only improved my skin health but also felt a deeper connection to the planet and the people around me," Emily shares. Her story is a powerful reminder that small, conscious decisions can lead to significant change. Through her journey, Emily became part of a larger movement toward a more sustainable and equitable future, proving that individual actions, no matter how small, can make a meaningful impact.

Key Takeaway

This journey of eco-conscious skincare is an ongoing process of learning, growth, and self-discovery. Embrace the challenges, celebrate your successes, and continue to strive towards a more sustainable and fulfilling future. Remember, every small step you take, from choosing sustainable ingredients to sharing your knowledge with others, contributes to a larger movement towards a healthier planet and a more just and equitable world.

This is more than just a personal journey; it's about recognizing our interconnectedness with the planet and the collective impact of our choices. Every conscious decision we make, from the products we choose to the actions we take, contributes to a larger movement towards sustainability.

Individual Choices Matter:

Choosing sustainable products, minimizing waste, and supporting ethical brands may seem like small actions, but they have a significant collective impact.

By making conscious choices in our daily lives, we demonstrate our commitment to a more sustainable future and inspire others to do the same.

A Collective Responsibility:

We share a collective responsibility to protect our planet and ensure a healthy and sustainable future for generations to come.

By working together, supporting sustainable businesses, advocating for change, and inspiring others, we can create a powerful movement that drives positive change and contributes to a more just and equitable world.

This journey of eco-conscious skincare is not just about achieving healthy skin; it's about embracing a holistic approach to well-being that considers our impact on the planet and contributes to a more sustainable future for all.

Conclusion

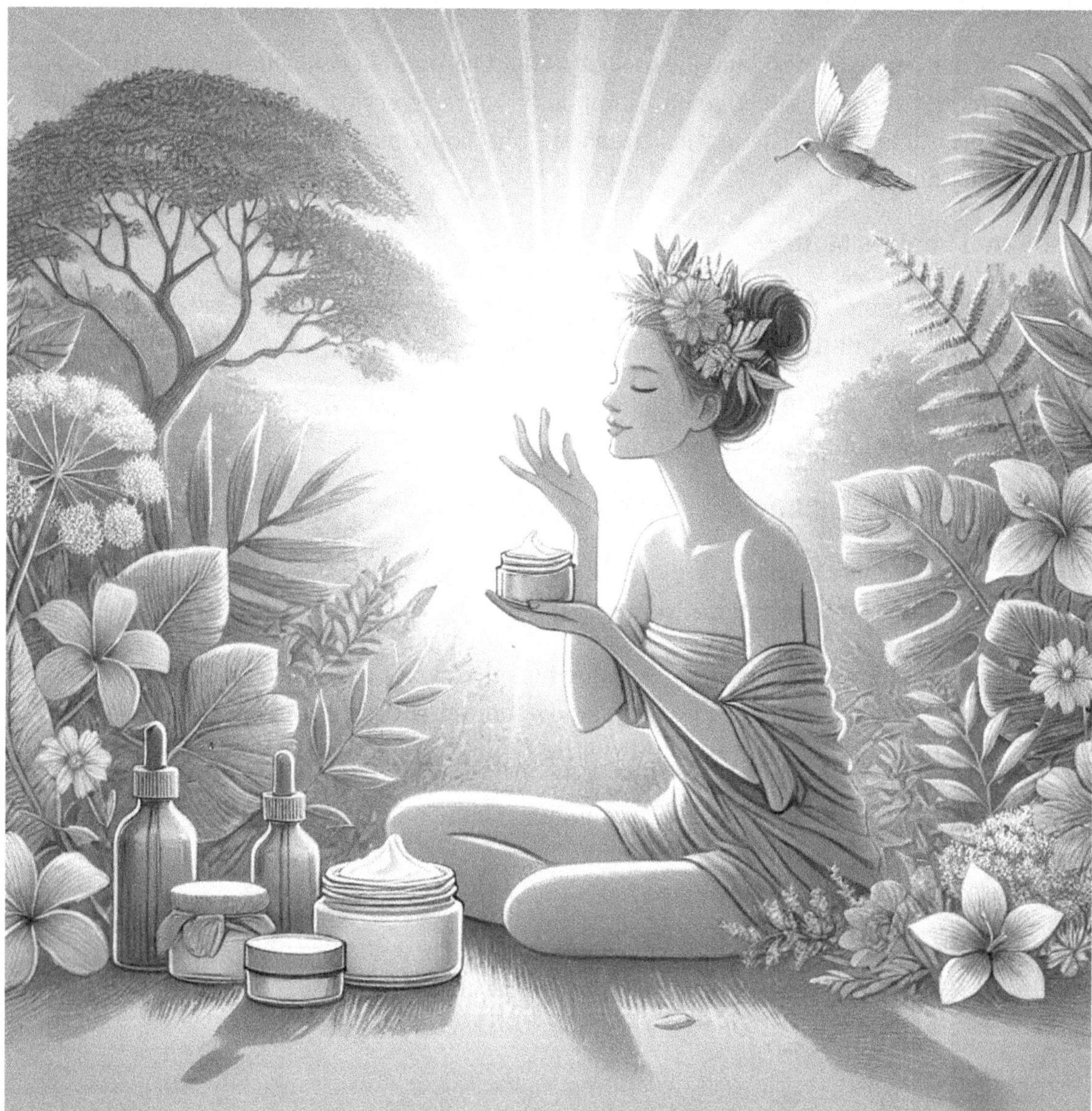

As we conclude this journey together, I encourage you to embrace the power of conscious choices and the transformative potential of eco-friendly skincare. Remember, this is not just about creating beautiful skin; it's about creating a beautiful and sustainable future for ourselves and generations to come.

Big Thank You

Thank you for embarking on this journey with me. I hope this book has inspired you to embrace eco-friendly skincare, nurture your skin, and contribute to a healthier planet.

Further Reading and Resources

Books:

"The Skin Care Bible" by Paula Begoun

"The Chemistry of Cosmetics" by Harry B. Brock

"The Complete Herbal Handbook for Vibrant Health" by Rosemary Gladstar

"Sustainable Style" by Lauren Singer

Websites:

Environmental Working Group (EWG): https://www.ewg.org/

The Good Trade: https://www.thegoodtrade.com/

Project Drawdown: https://drawdown.org/

Organizations:

Surfrider Foundation: https://www.surfrider.org/

World Wildlife Fund (WWF): https://www.worldwildlife.org/

Greenpeace: https://www.greenpeace.org/international/

Disclaimer

This book is for informational purposes only and should not be considered medical advice. The information provided in this book is based on the author's research and personal experience and should not be considered a substitute for professional medical or dermatological advice.

Always consult with a qualified healthcare professional before making any significant changes to your skincare routine or if you have any concerns about your skin health.

This book may contain information about herbs, plants, and other natural substances with potential health benefits. However, it is crucial to understand that these substances may interact with medications, cause allergic reactions, or have unintended side effects for certain individuals, including pregnant or breastfeeding women.

The author and publisher assume no responsibility for any adverse effects that may result from the use of the information or recipes contained in this book.

This book is not a substitute for professional medical advice: It's crucial to consult with a healthcare professional for any specific skin concerns or before making significant changes to your skincare routine.

Potential interactions with medications: Some natural ingredients may interact with medications you are currently taking.

Possible side effects: Natural ingredients can cause allergic reactions or other side effects in some individuals.

Disclaimer of liability: The author and publisher are not responsible for any negative outcomes resulting from the use of the information provided in this book.

Copyright Information